Joyce Delaney works in a large hospital in the English Midlands. She started to write a few years ago and published a novel, *Come Down From the Mountain*. Then followed her very successful autobiographical books *No Starch In My Coat, Smile at Me Doctor* and *Pass The Happy Pills**. Her uneasy dedication to Medicine continues to endure and she is fascinated by doctors and patients, their faults and virtues and the dearth of bores amongst them.

Joyce Delaney feels that the one great legacy given to her by a convent education is a sense of discipline which enables her to have a full-time job, run a house and find time for writing. She is a regular contributor to *World Medicine*, and broadcasts on occasions.

*Also available in Sphere Books

D1556624

It's My Nerves, Doctor

JOYCE DELANEY

SPHERE BOOKS LIMITED
30/32 Gray's Inn Road, London WC1X 8JL

First published in Great Britain by Sphere Books Ltd 1980
Copyright © Joyce Delaney 1980

TRADE
MARK

Set in Lasercomp Baskerville

Printed and bound in Great Britain by
Collins, Glasgow

IT'S MY NERVES, DOCTOR

Chapter One

When I was a young doctor I was so tuned in to night calls that I woke with the speed of a well-conditioned laboratory rat when the phone rang in the small hours. But, as I grew older, it was hellish trying to wake, trying to ease myself out of a sleep which was the more prized because it was hard to come by. But this Sunday night I wasn't even on duty. And it was nearly Monday morning, too. I grabbed the phone crossly, the apprehension of bad news putting a frost on my voice.

'Yes?'

'Oh. It's Paddy Moore here. Remember me?'

Would I ever forget? Paddy was a very bright young man whose genius in passing examinations was equalled only by his self-destructiveness. Three times he'd come into hospital and we'd treated his wrecked body and mind, but he refused to go to a unit specially designed to help young addicts like him with long-term and intensive psychotherapy.

'I hope you don't mind me ringing you like this, Doctor?'

I was going to say that yes, I certainly did, when I thought of his history. Brought up to believe his mother was his sister and with no one, not even his mother, having a clue to who Paddy's father was, it wasn't strange that relationships were difficult and love impossible for him.

'Just wanted to tell you that everything is falling into place now, Doctor. I've been lying awake thinking all night and now things seem clear like.'

I wished I could say the same for myself. No wonder that even the Samaritans had got fed up with Paddy.

'What I'm going to do, Doctor, I'm going to go to that

unit we talked about. They've kept my place and I'm going to go there tomorrow. Oh, that's today isn't it?'

'That's right,' I said. I was glad to hear about his decision to go, I told him, but now I'd have to get some sleep.

'Yeah, yeah, well, just thought I'd let you know,' he said, and I put down the phone.

Of course sleep wouldn't come. I lay awake till dawn and then decided to get up. I set out for the hospital at about half past eight. It was always good to get to the hospital early on Monday mornings and this particular morning was still cool but with the promise of heat to come. We'd been enjoying a freakish spell of good weather for early May and the forecasters assured us of more. Normally Yorkely, the Lowry-like industrial northern town where I worked, was grey and dreary but now the sunshine made you forget the slag heaps, rearing chimneys and deserted mills.

Barrington Hall, the large psychiatric hospital where I was a consultant, still looked precisely what it used to be; a workhouse. Its narrow windows, from which the bars had only recently been removed, were grim and many of the older Yorkely residents still spoke of the 'Barrington Workhouse'. To them a suggestion of going there struck chill horror. But lots had been done with painting and decoration, and now even the long stone corridors seemed less daunting with pastel coloured walls. Cars, motorbikes and vans were drawing up outside and from them spilled the students, the psychologists, the social workers, physiotherapists, all the new young people who were doing so much to lighten and improve the bleak image of the hospital. At one time I knew all the staff but now they were changing so quickly that I only spotted a few that I knew.

Mrs Bell, my secretary, dashing between four phones handed me a sheaf of messages.

'Old Mrs Jardine is on about family poisoning her. Doctor would like you to see.'

'Mrs Taylor wants to know why GP has given her different pills from the ones you ordered?'

'Sue Begley wants to see you at the clinic because she saw a TV programme on phobias last night and wonders why you haven't put her on the treatment mentioned.'

I dealt with the queries although the weekend's business meant that all the GPs' lines were continuously engaged. The sick and bankrupt Health Service of 1978 didn't run to the six consultants at Barrington having a private office each. Post next. Mrs Bell had filtered the sheaf of mail for me and I slipped the bills into my bag and tried to dictate above the jangling phones. I had just managed to finish my letters when Doctor Hamil's surgery rang with a request for me to see that afternoon, a young man called Gary Timson at my clinic in St Basil's, the nearby general hospital. All right, I said, but would Mrs Bell inform Sister Morgan, the out-patient Sister there, about him?

Eleven o'clock. Now I had to visit both of my new-admission wards, Flower and Gilbert. They were used for patients who would stay no more than six weeks at the most. One patient in Flower Ward had had a bad weekend at home and had to be seen, two other patients felt so ill that they couldn't venture on a weekend out and wanted to talk to me. A sad girl with crippling anxiety had collapsed with fright in a lift in Yorkely. She took me a long time and I hadn't as many minutes to give as I'd have liked to a very depressed patient who'd been upset by her alcoholic husband calling her a 'nutter'. Fortunately, there were only a few routine problems in Gilbert Ward where my male acute patients were, and then I headed for my four 'long-stay' wards. They were full of geriatric patients and those tragic souls who'd become ill before the new drugs were introduced and who were either too institutionalised to be discharged or had no relatives able or willing to cope with them.

No time for lunch so I drove to St Basil's, resolving to try for an assistant. I'd had 'no' for Doctor Gupta, my nice Indian who had gone back to her own country six months ago. If I had someone working with me, taking over the long-stay wards and coming to the clinic with me, I could maybe have lunch sometimes and thus stop making a pig of myself eating junk food when I came home ravenous in the evenings. Better nobody than a dud, fair enough, but no harm in getting applications and possibly landing someone reasonable. If you didn't try you got nothing.

Sister Morgan, a blade-thin Scot, was hauling hopelessly at the awful window in my clinic room. We could never get it right. The room was too cold in winter and in heat like today, a stuffy inferno. All the complaints and requests Sister Morgan sent in produced nothing. Somehow her battle for air seemed to her to sum up what was wrong with the National Health Service. Surgeons had to wait years for a hook to hang their gowns on, the mortuary was filthy, and the attendants threatened to strike after a complaint, and one of the Sisters found nobody would serve her in the hospital canteen because she'd been heard to grumble about the patients' food being cold by the time it reached the ward.

'Best I can do, Doctor Delaney.' Morgan, her long face creased with tiredness, straightened her small white cap and hitched up her belt. No use hoping something would be done to give the room more ventilation, she said in the tones of someone defeated by bureaucracy and red tape. Like far too many Trojan workers she was counting the days to her retirement.

'There's young Gary Timson first,' she said bustling out her uniform crackling with starch.

He came in smoking. Punk hair style, earring in one dirty ear and wearing black leather. There was a badge with 'Try Me' on it pinned in his lapel. It seemed to sum up his air of cheeky aplomb.

'Don't know how you stand this room. It's like a bloody oven.'

He eased his collar while I scanned Dr Hamil's letter which wasn't at all informative. 'Says he gets tense as if he was going to explode and all the time he is worrying and unable to meet or mix with people.'

'Are you going to psycho-analyse me?' he asked, as I shifted in the cheap plastic chair which was stuck to my bottom.

'Let's find out the real problem first,' I said. 'What is your trouble, Gary?'

He stubbed out his cigarette and I saw the letters L-O-V-E tattooed on four of his stubby fingers. 'That's what I come to find out, in't it?' He shoved a stick of gum in his mouth and chewed ruminatively.

Oh, one of those, I thought. I could have reminded him that I'd fitted him in as a favour, that he hadn't an appointment, but I knew it would be no use. In his plastic world I was a psychiatrist, the new folk hero who was supposed to work the miracles that God used to perform, only He couldn't now because in Gary's terms God didn't, had never, existed.

The family history? Previous illnesses? After fifteen minutes Gary had lit another cigarette and I had only gleaned that his sister had asthma, his father had died in early life and his mother was doing three jobs and never at home. Schooling, how about that? I asked.

'Proper old load of rubbish they gave us there. Waste of time. Course, when I went to the Approved School I learned a few things,' he smirked.

'Why were you sent to an Approved School?'

'Well, I had to, didn't I? I was caught stealing a car along with a few other things I done with the gang. I had the social worker, the probation officer and two psychologists working on me. It was great. They was a great bunch of lads at the

Approved School and that's where I learnt me trade.'

His trade? I'd thought he was unemployed except for a brief spell of a few months as casual labourer.

'What is your trade, Gary?' I asked.

He transferred the gum from one bulging cheek to another. 'I'm a burglar,' he said, with the triumphant air of a Bugsy Malone.

I could feel sweat forming snakes down my face. I tried shifting my chair to get some respite from the glare of the window. Gary stared at me impassively, almost pityingly.

'It's a bugger that window. You want to get something done about it.'

'Have you . . .' I sought for the words. 'Done much burgling' or 'done any big jobs' sounded wrong, so I said, 'You mean you've made your living by burgling?'

'I told you, didn't I?'

'Are you in trouble now?'

'I'm due in court a fortnight today, aren't I? The police have it in for me see, what with me record and that.'

So that was it. He was fly enough to know that it might be worth trying to get a sympathetic psychiatric report to be read out to the court. Maybe that, too, was part of the training at the Approved School.

'Yeah,' he said. 'I got done for breaking and entering.'

Gary and I were never going to establish a rapport. Why hadn't he told Doctor Hamil about this?

'He never asked did he? Anyway, the bloke don't speak English right. He's a real Ying Tong like. Anyway, even if they send me down I don't mind doin' me porridge, it'll give me fiancay a chance to save. And with me nerves bad and that, I can be sent to the hospital during me stretch.'

Before I got him to give me more details of his absurd 'nerves', I found out more about his burgling career. He'd been in prison twice before, that was after some time in Borstal, and his previous brushes with the law were because of stealing a car, breaking into a factory and also some houses in Honeyacre, the rich part of Yorkely. He told me about the break-ins with bravado, dwelling on each as if they were proud notches on his gun, a proof of his virility and manhood. Grievous bodily harm and mugging were for the real yobs, not the Raffles figure which Gary seemed to think he was, putting himself on a high echelon of prestige in the underworld.

But his nerves, how did he consider he had nerves? Although I knew there were two new patients waiting outside, and I hated keeping new patients waiting because they were usually so strung up that a wait was horrific for them, Gary's preposterous boasting had a sort of social fascination. So, prison was the 'in' thing with trendy youth? I didn't hear much about drugs now, and sexual exploits were done to death, so maybe lads like Gary thought that gaols went with the Punk era.

'You wanted to know about me nerves like. Well, I get dizzy, fall about like, and me heart starts pounding. Then me insides churn and I come over all queer. Mum used to have nerves, see. Me face goes all red like hers used.'

Yes, and his description of what he imagined to be 'nerves' sounded as unlikely as his mother's menopausal flushes which, I imagined, gave him his idea of what mental illness was. He had no psychiatric symptoms I said firmly, none at all, and sorry, I couldn't give him any more of my time. I could have said that it was a wonder his victims didn't have nerves when they were burgled and that surely they were entitled to pity and attention. I had no intention of writing to any court and it was up to him to decide whether he was going to give up crime or take the consequences.

'I'll write to Doctor Hamil and tell him that you have no sign of any mental illness and don't require any psychiatric help,' I said firmly.

'What do you mean?' the baby face twisted, snarled and became very nasty. 'You never examined me. Never sounded me, not nothing.'

'I've been watching you, observing you for nearly an hour and carefully listening to everything you've said.' I tried to keep my voice as professionally cool as possible, and it was quite a job because I was beginning to get very tired of Gary with his non-problems. 'You probably cause other people to feel nervous,' I went on. 'Breaking into houses and frightening people.' God, I hoped he didn't find out that I lived on my own and burgle me!

'Listen,' he shouted. 'I come here for help. What about them shaking turns I get? And I 'eave after meals. And I don't sleep.'

'Then take up something else other than a life of crime,' I said. 'Now I have to get on with my work.'

'Bleedin' 'ell,' he shouted, getting up. 'Me mates told me I'd get 'elp from you but you're kicking me out! It's us who pays your bloody wages you know.'

I thought he was going to hit me and I prepared myself to say that if he didn't leave quietly I'd send for the police. But I didn't have to say anything. He deflated fairly rapidly and became wheedling. Couldn't he have a few 'sleepers' to keep him going? His 'fiancay' didn't like the Pill and would I fix her up with something else?

He must have seen by my face that there was nothing doing because he got up and said as a parting shot at the door, 'I'm going to report you. I'll tell my Probation Officer about you, that's what.'

He could do as he liked, I said, and he shot out slamming the door.

Morgan burst in straight after him. She looked like a cross horse. 'That laddie looks as if demons are chasing him. I had to check him twice for smoking while he was waiting, and the lip he gave me!'

'Me, too,' I said. 'He's a burglar, a nervous burglar.'

Morgan huffed and puffed in amazement, asking, 'What were things coming to when criminals came to clinics and took up our time? You know the girls in Casualty are asking

8

for police protection on Saturday nights. It's so rough. Why was the lad sent to you? Why shouldn't rogues like him face the law?'

He was going to, I said, but probably thought it was worth a try on with me first. GPs were too busy sometimes to take proper histories and the courts were snowed under by the increasing number of criminals they had to deal with, many of whom were truly mentally ill, to be sure, and should be accommodated in mental hospitals. The irony was that the psychiatric hospitals had all opened their doors, becoming as liberal and permissive as the progressives wanted, and thus were unable to accommodate the very disturbed criminals.

'The prisons are crammed to a dangerous level and there's been a move by the Government to try to establish regional secure units for housing the criminally insane, but nobody wants to know,' I said.

'Quite right, too. I'm sure if they wanted to build a regional secure unit on the estate where I live, all us residents would have something to say,' Morgan added.

That was the general reaction, I said. Meanwhile judges made scathing comments when mental hospitals refused to take patients who posed security problems, and the nursing unions stipulated that a potentially violent patient had to be assessed and vetted by a team of nurses before the patient was admitted.

It was almost a relief to deal with people who were psychiatrically ill after the tussle with Gary, and I even forgot about the heat and the stuffiness of the room as I got through the patients. The new patients were so ill that it didn't take much time to deal with them. One was a housewife, a depressive who hadn't taken her medication because she thought it was making her fat, deluded into thinking that she was a creature from outer space. She was psychotic enough to be wearing what she called her astral hat and moon boots. She hadn't refused to be admitted and her distracted husband would drive her to Barrington Hall right away. The other new patient was a quiet, introverted man who just hadn't been able to come to terms with his wife's slow death from cancer. He wanted to argue with me that surely he could now exercise freedom, have the final liberty of joining his wife? I might have been disposed to argue with him if I didn't know that he'd always been subject to depression, because his wife had been a patient of mine during a minor crisis in her life. Come in, I said to him, come into hospital for a spell and we'll treat your depression and if after that you still want to kill yourself, then that's your prerogative. That surprised him, he had thought that all suicides were thought to be mentally ill. Not so, I said, suicide could at times be the product of a very clear mind, but he was emotionally exhausted and so not able to make a rational or wise decision.

It was after five o'clock when my last patient left but now there were the overdoses to see. Morgan, dashing around with the energy of a woman half her age, paused for a moment and said,'What you need is an assistant. All the other doctors have one. The other consultants, I mean.'

I had to agree. By seven o'clock though, after seeing the ward patients, I still felt quite refreshed, probably by the many cups of tea I'd had during the clinic, and not yet ready to go back to the flat. It was the top part of a house called the Priest's House, presumably for the chaplain when the hospital patient population required a resident clergyman. It was situated a nice distance from Barrington, not too far and not too near, and I had it for a peppercorn rent. Every year I decided that I really must buy a house and not wait till I was too old to get a mortgage, but because I had my flat almost rent free and because it was so near the hospital, and the large gardens front and back were maintained for me, I always put things off, stuffing the idea of moving to the very back of my mind.

The Priest's House had another great advantage for me

It was only five minutes from Garland House where my friend Doctor Frankie Mullen lived with Barney Osborne who owned the house. Frankie and I had been students together and her friendship had helped brighten a time when I had no money, no confidence and no faith in the future. Frankie hadn't any money either because her father was a poacher in some remote country town and it was her mother who financed Frankie with her teacher's salary, which was pathetically puny. The difference though was that Frankie had every confidence in herself and in the future which didn't, she said, lie in medicine. I was delighted when I heard that, because I myself couldn't see any future in doctoring, none at all. I only carried on with it because my doctor father would have a fit if I didn't. No need to worry about that, Frankie told me, we'd both get married for sure. She stuck to this idea in spite of our lack of partners to take us to dances and having to suffer the humiliations of dates who didn't turn up, or if they did turned up drunk. We were wasted on bog-trotting students, Frankie said, they were too coarse and crude to appreciate women like us. Oh no, there had to be a Mr Right out there somewhere who would suddenly arrive and sweep us off our feet. We used to watch the other students bent over their dissections discussing which speciality they'd settle for, listen to them planning their careers, while Frankie and I egged each other on in our wildly romantic way. Slowly and horribly it dawned on us in our final year that we'd have to settle for a medical career if we were to eat while Mr Right was arriving.

But we both did get married some two years after qualifying. The only thing was that my marriage ended in an early divorce and Frankie's in early widowhood. I had one child, a son, and she had none.

'You'd have thought we'd be so fertile,' Frankie sighed when I met up with her again when she came to do a locum in Barrington Hall, 'that we'd have lashings of kids between us. Here we are, two people who were all set for marriage and kids, yet we end up like this. I suppose it's a good job we have our careers.'

Mr Right hadn't turned up for me and now I was realising that I was no Mrs Right myself! But it was lovely meeting Frankie again after the years apart whilst I had been abroad and she doing jobs in the North of England. She was as ebullient and vital as ever, even though her marriage, from her few remarks about it, hadn't been happy and her husband, a charming Scots doctor, had been a paid up member of the Alcoholic Club. 'A walking gin bottle,' as Frankie called him.

She'd tried her hand at all sorts of jobs from paediatrics to anaesthesiology and had decided that general practice was the job for her. Psychiatry didn't appeal to her at all.

'So many of the patients just need a kick in the pants,' she said. 'But maybe you're suited to it. It's better than working in a leper colony.'

I wasn't sure I liked that remark but my fondness for her overcame resentment, and I was glad she was staying on in Yorkely. This decision was due to her meeting someone when she did a stint in private practice in the town's salubrious residential area, Honeyacre. She got off the mark with a man called Barney Osborne who moved to Garland House after retiring from the army in India. Never a man to reveal his age, I'd put him in his early sixties and on bad days he could look eighty. They were both emotionally volatile and fiery personalities, kind and generous and sufficiently fond of each other to keep the stormy relationship going, in spite of the many eruptions between them. They'd rather, in fact, be sparring with each other than living in solitary dullness. They both had a quirky sense of humour which helped them to put up with each other. It was an odd, off beat sort of relationship, with no mention of marriage but they'd been living together in Garland House for five years now, ever since Frankie had gone into general practice in the neighbourhood. Her partner had died and she carried on single-handed till she got a young assistant.

Barney was made more irascible by a form of deafness which he'd had for some ten years. He used the condition ruthlessly to get his own way, even referring to it as 'My Affliction'. Deaf he was to some exent and the condition was indeed resistant to treatment. Maybe that was why he was so very anti-doctor, because although he was a great hypochondriac he couldn't stand the medical profession and never lost an opportunity to get in a dig at them.

As I was driving away from St Basil's I decided to call and see Frankie and Barney. I realised that Frankie wouldn't be back from her evening surgery but Barney would be there, delighted to have company. Due to a life spent, in the main, abroad, his deafness and an alarming touchiness which concealed shyness, Barney was a lonely man, more especially since Old Sullivan, the retired lawyer with whom he had played chess, had died a year ago.

Garland House was a spacious Georgian residence, a bit dilapidated outside and untidy within, but Frankie had done things with erratic decoration, and using her sharp eye at auctions to pick up the odd bit of Sheraton and Chippendale, had made the old house attractive and comfortable in a warm sort of way. And Barney matched his charming house. He had flops of very white hair, blue eyes which glittered electrically and a figure which, he was proud to point out, hadn't altered since his army days. Frankie told me he exercised regularly every morning and took care of his smooth pink skin by using a special vanishing cream which he ordered from London. He was a vain man and Frankie had never got over the time when during one of their most ferocious rows, she'd caught him studying his profile in the mirror over the mantelpiece.

This evening he was at his most gracious, an example of the thing Frankie admired most about him, his style or cavalry spirit, whatever you liked to call it. Frankie was a great snob probably because of her father's occupation, and I think she saw in Barney the epitome of the Anglo-Irish who lived in The Big House and who produced warrior scions to serve the Empire. She could be very cutting to Barney about what she called his out-of-date and tarnished views on everything and he, like her, was a great believer in free speech. Secretly though, she admired his being a gentleman and there was no one more interested than she when, if he was in the mood, he'd produce his photograph albums and mull over the lovely sepia shots of balls and shoots and hunts, all the gracious social events before the regiment pulled out of India.

Once, as she stared at a photograph of Barney, a young, golden god clad in his tennis whites and about to serve, she turned to me and said with great seriousness, 'Don't you think there's something, well, *noble* about Barney's face?'

Now, Barney was very much the host. He inspected his drinks table and asked me what I'd like. I settled for a glass of chilled white wine and sat happily in one of the battered but very comfortable leather arm chairs which, with the settee, had been in Barney's bungalow in India. He brought me my drink followed by Willy, his aged dog, who now spent most of his time sleeping.

While Barney fixed himself a drink, I sipped my wine and looked out through the open french windows on to a riotous garden which Barney looked after. Frankie had been forbidden to go near it after she'd dug up some very expensive plants that he had put in the day before. But she'd left her mark on the sitting-room, where we now sat. An enormous vase of flowers was placed on one of the half-moon tables and was reflected by the huge mirror that nearly covered one wall; the other was fitted with shelves of books, shabby from use because both Barney and Frankie were voracious readers. Barney was musical and when the mood took him, he'd tinkle for hours on the grand piano in the corner. It was a disappointment to him, he once told me, that Frankie had such vulgar and philistine tastes in music. It was even more of a disappointment that his deafness precluded him from going to concerts and the opera. He'd always relied on music and had never been lonely, no matter how remote his station, when he'd had his gramophone and radio.

It was a good thing he could read, he told me sadly as he sipped his drink. Days were long when you weren't working and gardening made a welcome occupation, but you could only do so much. Sitting up very straight, blue eyes staring into the distance, I could sense that he was going to indulge himself in a bit of self pity, so when he unexpectedly asked me just exactly how I filled *my* day, I took him up on it to avoid what Frankie called Barney's Poor-Little-Me mood.

'I know you work in Barrington Hall as a psychiatrist but I was rereading Freud all last week and it occurred to me to ask you what exactly a modern psychiatrist does. I know, of course, that you don't sit behind the patient with a note book, but what exactly *does* . . . a latter day . . .' He searched for the words.

'You want to know what a jobbing psychiatrist living in today's world does?' I prompted.

That was it, said Barney getting up to help himself to another drink.

While he twiddled irritably with the hearing aid which was the bane of his life, I explained that psychiatry had changed dramatically in the last twenty years, ever since the introduction of the Mental Health Act of 1959 which almost gave a charter of freedom to mental patients, opening doors and reserving the 'committal' or legal incarceration of patients in large institutions like Barrington, to the few and increasingly fewer patients who would not come in informally. Previous to the new charter mental illness was treated with the cruel fear accorded to leprosy. The insane were sent to the old workhouses or to Victorian monstrosities which were always tucked away in remote places for fear of offending the general populace. There were no real treatments other than padded cells, seclusion and restraint. Custodial care of the crudest sort was all that was available till the turn of the century. No wonder mental illness was tantamount to a death sentence, because very few of the unfortunates admitted to the barrack-like institutions ever got home again or, in some cases, ever received a visit from their relatives.

But where did Freud, Jung, Adler, all the great innovators come in? Barney asked.

The beginning of the century was a time of massive activity for psychiatry, I went on. The great pioneers he'd mentioned, Freud and the others, produced new and merciful explanations of mental illness. There was a tremendous amount of study and research done on the most neglected patients in medicine and, at last here was progress. Then the drug era began and psychiatry, having been opened up and studied with the respect due to an authentic field of medicine, became classified into illnesses which could at least be treated, even latterly, prevented. At last doctors stopped thinking of mental illness as the domain of clinical duds. The speciality began to attract psychologists, social workers and other trained and skilled people. The mental hospital actually began to discharge patients, having to readmit them sometimes, but at last being able to offer hope and a chance of resuming normal life. Newer and better drugs were coming out all the time. The stigma of mental disorder had all but gone, and there was a proliferation of hostels, half-way houses, day centres, night centres and community centres all with the aim of helping to keep a discharged psychiatric patient within the comminity. The aim nowadays was prophylactic, trying to *prevent* mental illness happening rather than treating it when it did. When I came to Barrington Hospital ten years ago it had a thousand in-patients, now there were less than half that number, and with the appointment of four community nurses and the establishment of all the out-patients at St Basil's, the hospital bed occupancy was steadily decreasing.

'But what about the really mad, the disturbed, type of patient?' Barney asked.

Infrequently we had to admit a patient against his will, to 'commit' him in fact, but it seldom needed to be for long and as for his being 'disturbed' well, we had such a wide variety of drugs now that it was simply a question of stabilising the patient on the drug which suited him best. Like diabetics whose lives were dramatically changed by insulin, our very disturbed patients who would formerly have been classed as 'mad' and dumped in a mental hospital, were now taking their place in the community on their regime of long-acting psychotropic drugs. We in the hospitals were increasing our work in the community, trying to link up with the social workers who were doing the same. Of course, treatment of patients within the community often placed great stress and strain on the community who had found things were easier when their psychotic relatives were tucked away in locked wards.

'I see. I see the progress, the changes, but tell me exactly what you do, an example of your day,' Barney said.

'First,' I said, 'you have to understand that every mental hospital serves a particular area, called a "catchment area". Barrington Hall serves an area ten miles in radius. There are six consultants and we have a rota, taking it in turns to be on duty for our catchment area. That means that one week in every six I'm on duty and have to take all the calls and emergencies from the catchment area, going out on visits, called "domiciliary visits", at the request of the patient's GP. As for my actual day, the best thing is to describe today . . .' Which I then did, leaving out the bit about Gary Timson because I knew it would only inflame Barney into a passionate diatribe on bringing back flogging.

The door crashed open and Frankie appeared. 'What a day,' she gasped, flinging down her shoulder-bag which bulged with her stethoscope. Everyone had decided to collapse and all the kids seemed hell bent on swallowing coins and sticking things up their noses. A midwifery case had turned so nasty that the woman had to be admitted to St Basil's, and she'd just come from a road accident near her surgery after which the bodies had almost to be scraped up.

'Ditto,' I said. 'I've just been telling Barney about my day.'

'Oh, really?' she said politely, but I knew she didn't believe we knew what hard work was in psychiatry. To Frankie's robust view the psychiatrists did too much hand holding with their patients and made them worse.

She sipped the wine Barney handed her, while he poked at the open fire with the old dress sword he used for the purpose. The fire was a source of continued friction between them. Barney claimed that anything but natural heat made him feel ill and that as his blood was thinned from the tropics he needed the warmth of a coal fire even on the hottest day. Frankie thought that in that case he should damn well clean and set the fire himself on the days the cleaning woman didn't come in. But Barney was of the generation holding the view that cleaning out grates was strictly women's work. Now, Frankie sat glowering at Barney as he rattled irately at the fire trying to coax the recalcitrant ashes to a blaze. Any minute now Frankie would bound up and heave at the fire with a poker, all the time grumbling about doing dirty, outmoded work.

She sat dark and smouldering, drinking her wine with quick, irritable sips. The rather massive handsomeness of her youth better suited her middle age. It was as if she'd grown into herself. The dark, white-streaked hair was drawn back in a tumbling chignon, her nearly black eyes were still bold and shiny and although her teeth were definitely crooked and her nose hooked, the general effect, due to her crackling vitality and élan, was of a comely woman. She could always wear bright colours which would look garish on other less vibrant personalities and today she wore a suit of acid yellow.

By the way she was frowning and glaring at Barney, I knew that she was going to let fly at him, but he doubled up with a fit of coughing, spluttering and choking so violent that he alarmed Willy, who crept away. Barney went out, gasping that he was going to get a handkerchief.

'What do you think of him?' Frankie asked, and I told her he'd been in crashing form, very well indeed.

'Did he tell you he had a haemoptosis, coughed blood this morning?'

'No, he didn't, but couldn't that be due to the rupture of a small blood vessel caused by the coughing?' A common but not serious condition and nothing to worry about.

'No, it was a genuine haemoptosis,' Frankie said. 'I'll just have to try and get him to go to Harper, his GP. Or better, have Harper call here.'

Surely she was being a bit over anxious, I told her. I wouldn't worry about it. Not at all.

'Ah, yes,' she said. 'But then you didn't have a brother and sister who died of lung cancer.'

Chapter Two

Barney never spoke about the brother and sister who died, the memory was too painful, especially that of his sister whom he had adored. Frankie thought maybe his distrust and loathing of doctors was due to their being unable to help his sister. Barney was a great hypochondriac, especially now that he had little to do, his health was becoming his hobby. It was how she'd first met him, Frankie said, he'd come to her panicking about a sore throat.

'And nearly bit my finger off when I tried to examine him. Oh well, I'd better go and see to him.'

Barney reappeared, however, looking pale and shaken but not coughing now. While Frankie was all solicitude Barney stalked over and poured himself a large drink. Frankie exploded.

'Jesus, Mary and Joseph, you're the limit, Barney. You should leave off smoking and drinking until you've had a check up.'

'Who said anything about a check up?' Barney snarled and began to light a cheroot. Frankie let out such a shriek of horror that Barney dropped his match in fright on poor Willy's neck. The dog howled and fled under a chair while Frankie ranted at Barney for complaining about his health and blaming doctors for being no good, whilst he set about destroying himself with nicotine and alcohol.

'Christ, you'd think I was never sober to listen to you! Listen, my ear is buzzing. There are noises pulsating through my head with your shouting and screaming.'

Whilst he turned his back on her, Frankie appealed to me for support. I remained mute, too wise in the ways of my friends even to try to take sides.

Barney, almost frothing and in danger, I thought, of getting another coughing spasm with ill-temper, pointed his cheroot defiantly at Frankie and shouted furiously, 'Now get this, Frankie. I am going to continue the few pleasures that make my life bearable. No matter what you or Doctor Billy Harper say. I lead a sad and lonely life plagued by deafness, and you now seek to deprive me of the two anodynes that prevent me from committing suicide. Finish me off why don't you? Give me the injection I'm always asking for, but don't be so bloody petty as to take away the small bits of anaesthesia that help me to get through life. Not having pleasure mind, just hanging on.'

This was all vintage Barney. Well into his stride now, he shook his finger at Frankie yelling that it was all bloody fine for her, an aggressively healthy woman, he paused and emphasised the 'aggressively' for effect, and just because she herself had good health she ought, as a medical woman, to be able to sympathise with those like himself who hadn't.

'I bloody pity your unfortunate patients,' he roared.

I was afraid Frankie would rise to this bait but with a terrific effort, probably being as worried as I was by the panting heaves which were beginning again, she made her voice as sweet as she could and apologised to Barney, who grunted.

'It's all you doctors want to do, to terrify people about their cholesterol, the dangers of nicotine and the risk of pollution. No wonder Joyce tells us that people are having so many breakdowns.'

Frankie, keeping a grip on herself, said wasn't it time we ate? She'd make scrambled eggs, she said. They were Barney's favourite dish so I knew she was trying to placate him. I'd have to go, I said, and left the two of them exchanging pleasantries. It was nearly ten o'clock and my interrupted sleep of last night was catching up on me.

As I parked my car in the garage and walked around to

the back of the Priest's House I resolved to beard Felix Coulter in the morning. He was the Chairman of our medical committee and although he wasn't liable to help me get an assistant because he really didn't give a damn about anyone apart from himself, I could at least persuade him to put an advertisement in the journals.

I slept deeply and went to the hospital next morning feeling fine. It was becoming impossible to tell patients from staff but now I couldn't tell staff from staff. Two girls in blue denim pants and blouson tops were coming in with me. Their long hair swung around their earnest young faces and on their bare feet they wore rope mules.

'Hi!' one of the girls said to me, and it dawned who she was. Lee Kelly, the new psychologist.

Barney had asked me the difference between a psychologist, a psychiatrist and a psycho-analyst. A psychiatrist, I had told him, is a medical doctor who had an extra degree in psychiatry, a psycho-analyst could be a lay-person but was usually a psychiatrist and he specialised in giving psychotherapy, often based on the association techniques of Freud or Jung. But a psychologist, is a graduate in psychology only, not medicine, and does things like measuring intelligence and treating conditions like phobias by conditioning and retraining. To mention Freud to a bright, young member of a new speciality like psychology, was to risk being thought very old hat. To the psychologist behaviourism was the thing and they got mad if you told them, as I had once, that human beings were more than rats leaping about a box getting rewards and punishments. Well, maybe to the young life was a maze of complications, and with God now less than a music hall joke, possibly the rewards of a sweet and the punishment of an electric shock were the only operatives.

'Morning, Lee,' I said as the girl swung the fall of ash blonde hair from her face. She looked dewy and young without make-up.

'Oh, Doctor Delaney, I wanted a word with you. Remember Wendy Cotton, the girl you sent to me because she had a stammer?'

'Yes. Oh, yes,' I said, picturing the white-faced girl.

'Well, the stammer's gone. But now she's depressed and I'm a bit worried. Would you see her, please? As soon as possible?'

So Wendy's stammer had been helped. But as Freud had cogently noted, didn't the elimination of one symptom often cause the appearance of another? Useless to say things like that, thought, to this cool-voiced blonde with the air of calm reason.

'O.K. Tell Wendy to come to my clinic at St Basil's in two days' time.'

'Thanks. Oh . . . hi, Felix . . .'

Felix? I watched Doctor Coulter acknowledge the greeting by flipping a limp hand. He wore a lint coloured jacket and carried a briefcase. He liked to be trendy and his cheesecloth shirt and flourishing, fair side-burns were concessions to what he imagined was 'with it'.

'Could I see you for a moment, Felix?' I asked. Now was the time to grab him. I'd heard he was going away soon.

'Sure, sure. In my office,' he said, not looking at me.

While Coulter flipped through his mail I stood waiting. I'd got used to him not asking me to sit down; that sort of good manners was something he never bothered with. The big old room looking out on to the front avenue of the hospital had had a quite impressive character in the days of Doctor Samuel McKinnon, the last Superintendent of Barrington. The only remnants of that time ten years ago, before a massive coronary had carried McKinnon away, was the faded portrait over the heavy marble fireplace. I stared at the glowering and thunderous features of the old man. He reminded me, with his craggy nose and jaw and mutton chop whiskers, of pictures of Mr Gladstone. There was the same impression of Jove-like geriatric power. Some of the older nurses told stories of the way McKinnon would make his stately rounds, flanked by an entourage of senior nursing staff and the two medical officers which had made up the staff of a hospital of well over a thousand beds. There were anecdotes of the feudal way in which staff could be dismissed or 'sent down the avenue' as it was called, for minor offences, and the dread caused by an order to 'come to the Super's office'. Nearly as bad as a summons to Matron Hall's office. She was an enormous old lady who had never had any formal training, but who was able, by sheer steel of personality and Nightingale-like zeal, to rule her nursing empire as firmly as McKinnon his medical one. I had seen photographs of her with a bulldog look and a stumpy dignity reminiscent of Queen Victoria.

What would Matron and Doctor McKinnon think of things now? The in-patients cut to hundreds? Integrated wards, and nurses without uniform? Everybody eating the same food in the same canteen and all the erstwhile doctors' quarters made into offices for the administrators? No more patients' farm, laundry, or pools of patient labour for work in the senior staffs' rent-free houses. All the change and progress of the last ten to twenty years, with a huge and antiquated old building like Barrington costing a fortune to heat and maintain, and yet no money in the National Health kitty to level the place and start to erect a structure that was more in keeping with change and patients' needs. Trouble is, I thought, a hospital is out of date now before it's finished.

Coulter made a few phone calls and dictated some letters to his secretary, Mrs Watson, a most efficient little woman, in spite of her heavy hand with powerful scent which she once told me she used because of her fear of some lingering smell from the wards. She was in her sixties and probably imbued with the memory of paraldehyde which used to impregnate us all. She also wielded a blue rinse too heavily on her hair which sometimes could be a shade too azure, but she was a fast and vastly efficient secretary who maintained a discretion and decorum worthy of the highest civil servant in Whitehall.

Sun was beginning to flood through the windows. It was a room very suited to the colourless character of Coulter. No doubt about it. His arrival at the hospital ten years ago had coincided with a frenzy of decorative improvement, financed by a temporary influx of hospital funds. The jazzy curtains didn't suit the heavy bow windows at all and the carpet had a pattern which resembled squashed flies. The flat-topped desk didn't have anything like the noble proportions of the old mahogany one and the chairs, like most of the others in the hospital, looked cheap and plastic and felt sticky and uncomfortable.

'With you in a sec, Joyce,' Coulter murmured, sticking one of his innumerable cigarettes in his mouth. He was pacing up and down behind his gimcrack desk, puffing away and rattling loose change in his pocket.

Frankie and myself used to indulge in speculations about the Coulter character. What made him tick? Where, with his modest qualifications, was he going to? How indeed had he got where he was? Ever even qualified? But we hadn't allowed for his ambition and political nous. He hadn't done any good for the hospital but he'd made no enemies and kept his slate clean with the authorities. He was on at least ten committees and was adept at the boring jobs which nobody else wanted wanted. His very lack of personality kept him floating on top and there was never a breath of any scandal about him. Frankie had once had a theory that he might be homosexual as he seemed to enjoy being surrounded by good-looking and sycophantic young registrars, but even that idea seemed too positive after Mrs Coulter arrived. She was a large woman with a certain coarse, auburn beauty and Coulter was most uxorious and attentive to her. Her blazing hair and temper made him scurry to her side and Frankie said once that it was as if Maudie Coulter's flamboyant beauty attracted and held the albino-like Felix.

'Now then. Be with you in ten minutes Mrs Watson. And get me those memos, I want to take them with me.'

I'd just caught him, Coulter explained. He was chairing a meeting at Haxton Hospital which was outside London and a good two hundred miles away. Coulter's junketings narked us, the rest of the consultants. He seemed to be out of the hospital more than he was in it and this absence was due to his managing to get the pick of the young doctors working for him, all of them ready and eager to avail themselves of the medical patronage that Coulter handled so well. He mightn't be academic and certainly wasn't better qualified than the rest of us, but he had skill in making the most of what he had got. And that wasn't any more than tremendous energy. Frankie said you could add ambition.

As Coulter resumed his pacing I asked him whether the advertisement for an assistant for me had gone into the journals? Things were hard, clinics getting longer and there was my holiday to come.

'Aye. Never did replace Gupta did we?'

Coulter sounded a bit distant but not off-putting. In fact, now that I looked closer at him he looked positively jovial. He told me what I expected to hear of course, the lack of funds for medical staff, the dearth of suitable candidates and so on, but the expression on his pale and puffy face was quite genial.

'Leave it with me,' he said graciously. And that phrase deadened my hopes. All of us at Barrington knew that Coulter's 'leave it with me' was the kiss of death.

'It's not that I'm *asking* you for an assistant, Felix,' I said, stung into renewed action. 'I'm *telling* you that I must have help or else I'll have to write to the administration and let them get on with it.'

'I shouldn't think it'll come to that,' Coulter smiled placidly. Usually any mention of 'taking things further' caused him a furtive sort of panic which Frankie said was a crude and infantile fear mechanism. He pattered around the desk and ushered me out with a hand on my shoulder.

I walked along the corridor to my wards and nearly passed Tony Manners, one of the consultants.

'You look stricken,' he said. 'Sort of stunned. Have you had a tax rebate?'

I was still reeling after Coulter's warm reception I explained. Not that I was asking any favours. Only my rights. It was just that I hadn't expected Felix to be so receptive to my request for an assistant.

'You're not plugged in to the grapevine, dear. Haven't you heard our Felix might be going Stateside?'

'To America! But who . . .?'

'Who would take our Felix? Well, there's been some chap over from the States recruiting for a hospital there. He's a Professor Malone –his brother's a consultant at Haxton.'

'That's where Felix said he was going today.'

'Well. It all fits, doesn't it? Not that it'll make any difference to us, except that if Felix goes we can try to get another consultant who's not such a dead beat.'

I'd heard something about Coulter going I told Manners. But surely that had always been in the wind?

'The wind's getting stronger now though. Maybe Maudie Coulter's getting more impatient. I hear she's got very expensive tastes.'

Maybe the fact that Felix was surer of going to America meant that he was in better humour I pondered, as I walked up the corridor towards Gilbert Ward where I had my new male admissions. At least I'd stated my case instead of going around feeling aggrieved and hard done by.

'Good morning, Doctor.' Mr Latimer, the charge nurse, greeted me as he always did with hushed reverence.

Percy Latimer, the fortyish charge nurse, was about the only nurse left in the hospital who still wore a white coat and, not only that, he changed his coat twice a day, just as I was sure he polished his shiny boots (he never wore shoes), at least once in twenty-four hours. He was a burly man with slicked back hair glistening with Brylcreem, and rather bulging light grey eyes. He walked with the heavy stamping gait of an RSM and indeed he was never done telling us that his stint in the army was one of the happiest times of his entire life. Its order and regularity suited his obsessional character and one of his moans was that National Service had been abolished.

Mr Latimer grumbled a lot. He'd never come to terms with integrated wards, especially after working·for a short and disastrous period on one of them. A nubile female patient had propositioned him by lifting her skirt to reveal a plump, white thigh and Latimer had asked for an immediate transfer. He hated doctors without white coats and nurses with long hair. The first names tossed around so freely made him mournful and it was said that he'd never got over seeing Felix Coulter expend blow and spit, playing his saxophone in the Conservative Club.

'No decorum' was a favourite and much quoted phrase of Latimer's. Still, though short on humour, he was kind and concerned about his patients and spent time and trouble listening to them and getting to know them.

'A new admission to see, Doc,' Latimer puffed, as he pulled back a chair for me at the desk of the ward office. 'This lad, Ian Nelson, was admitted last evening after taking an overdose of lavatory cleaner washed down by whisky.'

Novel sort of overdose, I commented as Latimer chivvied up a young nurse who had appeared to fetch the patient.

'We haven't much on the lad, because his own GP was off duty and the Emergency Service had to deal with him.'

The Emergency Service was fine and meant more reasonable hours for GPs, but the information about patients could sometimes, as now, be deficient.

'Mrs Nelson, the mother, is here and would like to see you afterwards. I'm afraid I haven't got anything out of the patient myself because we had a burst in one of the pipes and it took me ever such a long time to get the plumbers. Sit down here, lad.'

The patient was about nineteen I guessed, and he was clean and scrubbed-looking in a white shirt and blue denims. His face was pale with washed-out blue eyes which had a dead, empty look.

I went over the early history. There wasn't any really. He'd been an only child but had a normal early life and he lived with his mother with whom he got on well, he said. All the time he spoke, his voice low and composed, he had a half smile on his face. He worked in a factory and, yes, he quite liked that.

'So. Up to the overdose things have been all right, Ian,' I said. 'What made you take the overdose then?'

'I just got fed up like. After the cat.'

'The cat? Was it a pet?'

'Not a pet. Me mother took it in as a stray. I just got fed up with the way it was always staring at me. I don't like animals anyhow and this moggie was a nasty piece of work. It bit me when I came home the other night.'

'So?'

'I wanted to teach it a lesson. I tried to put it outside but it bit me so . . .' He stopped and the half smile flickered. 'So I cut off its legs with shears.'

It was as if he was talking about something as ordinary as making a cup of tea. I could hear Latimer panting beside me. A cold blooded psychopathy like Nelson's always shocked me in the extreme; the deed was callous enough but the deadpan, chilly lack of emotion was yet more terrible.

'Ever done anything like this before?' I asked and the youth shrugged.

'Can't remember. Can I go home now?'

'Right now? With your mother?'

He nodded.

I told Latimer to let him get his things while I had a word with the mother. Latimer showed Nelson out then said,

'Nasty little bugger. Sorry, Doc. Never liked that sort of psychopath. He reminds me of a lad I saw some years ago who strangled puppies and ended up in the Old Bailey.'

Mrs Nelson was a wispy little woman who said that she was puzzled about her son's behaviour. He'd always been a well-behaved, quiet son, rather a 'loner' in fact, but never giving any trouble. She thought the overdose was probably due to Ian's having been abandoned by his girl-friend who, she said, was 'common' and a bad lot anyway. Mrs Nelson was far more concerned with the faults of the girl than her son's act of cruelty to the cat.

Had Ian ever been cruel to animals before, I pressed her?

'Did he tell you about the goldfish?'

'What about the fish?' I asked.

'Well. When Ian was about ten, his dad was alive then and him and me went out for a bevvy and we left Ian on his own. We had a goldfish then, and when we got back Ian was in bed and we found he'd stabbed the fish with a knife and the bowl was full of blood. Dad gave Ian a good old thumping and asked him why he done it, but Ian just said the fish was stupid and had made faces at him. Well, can I take him now, Doctor?'

What was the point in keeping him? Ian wasn't suffering from mental illness as such and a psychiatric hospital had nothing to offer a cold, sick personality like Ian Nelson. Especially when unaccompanied by remorse. I felt grim and sad about his future though.

I was kept pretty busy by calls for the rest of the day until I took a breather at four o'clock and was able to ring Frankie to ask how Barney had got on. I didn't expect her to be in but she told me she had taken the day off to go to see the doctor with Barney.

'He's examined him from top-to-toe and says all is well, but he's ordered an X-ray just the same . . .'

I could hear Barney playing the piano in the distance, always a good sign, and I had to shout to make myself heard above Barney carolling 'Tell me pretty maiden'.

'He's in powerful form as you can hear,' Frankie said.

Great news, I said. And I had a bit of good news myself. I told her about Coulter's comparatively warm reception and the rumour about his leaving.

'Then, my dear, you have *had* it. He was in good form because the future is looking bright for the Coulter fortunes, and he doesn't give one tuppeny damn for what happens to the hospital or you. I'm surprised you haven't twigged. An old campaigner like you.'

It hadn't been my day. Except for the fact that there had been no calls since the afternoon. I decided that things were too good to last and so they were, because shortly after midnight my phone shrilled, just after I had got to sleep.

Chapter Three

'Miss Pillsworth, social worker, here, Doctor. I'm afraid I've got a problem.'

Oh no! Not Kate Pillsworth, I thought as I heaved myself out of the comfort of deep sleep. Miss Pillsworth was trying enough during the day but at this hour . . .

'The patient is an Indian, Doctor, and apparently he was admitted to Barrington Hall yesterday but refused to stay and discharged himself. Now Doctor Khan, his GP, has sent a message to me to say that Mr Dippy, the patient, should go back to hospital.'

'What's the matter with Mr Dippy?'

'I don't know. He speaks no English and I don't know why he was sent to hospital in the first place.'

'What about asking Doctor Kahn?'

Or was that too simple, I felt like asking. She couldn't get Khan back, Miss Pillsworth said, because he'd gone out on another call but he'd promised to come along later.

'Could you come along to the house Mr Dippy's staying in? Where I am now.'

'What do you want *me* for?'

In case Mr Dippy needed to come back to hospital. In case there was a question of committal and using a Section of the Mental Health Act for which my signature would be necessary, Miss Pillsworth explained.

I wanted to say testily that she'd have been better advised to find out what exactly was wrong with Mr Dippy before phoning me. To contact me as a 'just in case' measure was the wrong way to tackle things. But I knew my Miss Pillsworth once she got her teeth into something, and from experience of her importunate and obsessional way of managing things, I caved in and told her I'd be along directly. She proceeded to give me complicated directions about how to find the boarding house where Mr Dippy dwelt, until I reminded her that I, too, had an A to Z map of the city.

Social Services were, on the whole, reasonable people full of admirable energy and enthusiasm They were mostly bright, young people whose university courses in sociology had made them keen to practise their convictions that if only people were able to get a decent social deal then everything would fall into place. Doctors seemed to them at first to be rather hierarchical and authoritative relics of the bad old 'Them' and 'Us' times and on occasion one got the impression that the feeling among social workers was that medicine was far too important to be left just to the doctors. This attitude made for less than harmonious relations at times. As one old GP had said to me recently, 'I've been in practice thirty-five years and it comes hard to have a young social worker tell me how to suck my medical eggs.'

But as in the case of young doctors, time and experience mellowed the social workers, and on the whole, they were helpful, and anxious to get involved in helping patients. After I'd got used to their jargon of calling patients 'clients' and referring to things like 'the multi-disciplinary team', my relations with them were cordial and, I liked to think, therapeutic. But Kate Pillsworth was something else. Oh, she was keen. And she was eager. That was just the trouble. Her undoubtedly high IQ and terrific social conscience was untempered by commonsense and nous. Several of Yorkely's GPs had complained about her and she had been the subject of a few irate letters, but Kate carried on in her clumsy way.

Mr Dippy's abode was deep in the sleazy part of the city, an area thickly populated with Indians and West Indians. The house was shabby and peeling and, as I was putting the crook-lock on the car, Miss Pillsworth loomed over me. She was very tall with a huge mop of frizzy, red hair which enveloped her pale, freckled face like a busby.

She was sorry to have to call me she said, leading the way into the house. But she couldn't get the facts about Mr Dippy and as Doctor Khan was held up she thought she ought to contact me.

'For a second opinion, as it were,' she said, clumping up the narrow stairs with a heavy tread. She had spent several hours with Mr Dippy and as he spoke no English and his friends' knowledge of the language wasn't much better, she felt that the whole matter needed investigation.

Why the hell had she called me without facts? Surely it would be better to wait and see what Doctor Khan had to say? I bit back my irritability as Kate flung open the door of a room on the fifth floor. As I stood panting and getting my breath back after our climb, Miss Pillsworth strode over to the small man standing near the window. He had on a small, black skull cap and he wore a baggy white tunic over his *dhoti*. As Kate explained in sign language who I was, the little old man threw me a terrified look and began to finger his wooden beads. There were six other Indians in the room in various states of undress. For an all-male establishment I was surprised at the cleanliness of the place. The beds were skimpy but neat, the floor covering was very old lino but it shone, and the shirts hanging up around the walls were spotless.

'He is praying for us all,' one of the Indians grinned. 'All the time he prays. Never stopping.'

Nothing so peculiar in that. What was mentally wrong with him?

That set off the rest of the men in a barrage of quick fire Indian-English of which I couldn't make out much except that poor Mr Dippy was 'crazy' and 'acted funny'.

'That's it, you see.' Kate sighed. She had sat down on one of the beds and was gazing around the group of Indians with a deeply serious expression. Flinging out her arms she made

34

several attempts to explain that as none of us knew how and why Mr Dippy had been sent to Barrington Hall, it was vital to find out just what the matter was.

'Why do you say Mr Dippy is mad?' I asked one of the men when I could make a break in the animated conversation.

'He's mad. Keeping praying all the time,' the man said, tapping his head significantly.

'In this country . . . in England . . . we have to be very careful about sending people into a mental hospital. Especially when they do not speak English,' Miss Pillsworth said earnestly. Her hair sticking out like a bronze aureole, she launched into a description of the Mental Health Act and the rights of the individual. Mr Dippy stood apart looking at her in terror and began to pray very loudly. His friends gathered around Miss Pillsworth and stared at her as if they were pupils and she the guru. Maybe she reminded them of the *mem sahibs* who were relics of the Raj.

Where was Doctor Khan? It was after two o'clock and as for me, I was more confused than ever. I whispered to Kate who said yes, so was she, and that was why she'd called me out. You had to be so careful in implementing the Mental Health Act, she went on. So strict in assessing patients and very vigilant and protective of an individual's rights. On and on she went about this until I could have screamed. I then felt ashamed, as I always did, about the rage she induced in me. It wasn't so much what she said as the governess tone she used and the self-righteous manner of the way she imparted her beliefs, as if I were a slow and rather dull child and she the enlightened teacher. While her rather equine face grew more and more earnest and her accent more didactic I tried to remember that she was young and inexperienced and would probably get her come-uppance one of these days!

It was better when Doctor Khan arrived at three o'clock, full of apologies for having been delayed by someone who had had a brain haemorrhage. He spoke Mr Dippy's dialect, which was lucky because apparently the little man came from a remote part of India and none of his friends could really understand him.

Mr Dippy and Doctor Khan began to talk together in an impassioned exhange and once or twice Doctor Khan threw back his head and laughed loudly. After twenty minutes Dippy looked less frightened and Khan turned to me.

'What you call a comedy of errors, Doctor. I myself wasn't involved with Mr Dippy's admission into Barrington but his experiences there were so traumatic that he is fearful of being sent back, and begs you to leave him alone. He is a very holy Muslim as you can see and he is only three months in the country. He is a bus driver and finds that his prayer time is interrupted by his job. Two days ago there was some incident in the bus and some youths became insolent and insulting to Mr Dippy. I do not know what exactly happened . . .' Khan laughed apologetically as if excusing his holy countryman. I was trying to figure how Dippy managed to do his job without any English and Khan continued, 'Starting from scratch, as it were, Mr Dippy felt the Prophet was being vilified so he got very agitated and very angry. The police were called and Mr Dippy was brought to the police station. Again, I do not know what happened but the police doctor sent Mr Dippy to Barrington Hall. There he received a number of nasty shocks. First of all he was sent to a mixed ward and, because he is not used to this mingling of the sexes, he was shocked to see ladies and gentlemen walking around in night attire. Then he was examined by a young lady doctor and worst of all –' Khan paused, '– worst of all he was given a *pork chop* for supper! So traumatised he was that he ran away from the hospital in his pyjamas and wandered on to the motorway where he was picked up by the police. He is now wondering whether you are going to send him back to somewhere he thinks of as hell.'

Poor Mr Dippy flung himself to the floor in front of me and began to pray with passionate intensity.

So he's not crazy? Should never have been sent to Barrington Hall? I asked.

While Mr Dippy intoned, Doctor Khan burst out laughing again although Kate Pillsworth looked at him reproachfully. No, no, Mr Dippy wasn't mad, Khan said, just terrified lest we send him back to hospital.

'Tell him we're not going to, and that he never should have been sent in the first place,' I said firmly.

While Doctor Khan reassured Dippy, Kate Pillsworth murmured how terrible it all was. We might as well be in Russia where innocent parties like Mr Dippy were incarcerated against their will. If the poor little man had any standing he'd go off and complain to his MP.

'Now I must go. I have yet two calls to make.' Khan whipped up his black bag and, laughing gaily, went off while all the Indians began to shake hands with Kate and myself.

'All this could have happened to my Uncle Joseph,' Miss Pillsworth said as we went downstairs. Uncle was a strict and very devout Catholic who spent his life going to Mass and saying various litanies and offices during the day. He was a simple and holy man of God, she went on, as we were shown out of the house by the many more Indian gentlemen who popped out from nowhere.

I had a job to break away from Kate who was now well and truly launched into a dissertation on human rights. She was justified. Poor Dippy had been victimised, was even due an apology which I knew he'd never get. If only Kate wouldn't keep on, not just making points, but ramming them home with furious tosses of her wild red hair.

'I'm sorry to have called you so late, Doctor, but I felt it was necessary,' she said, grabbing my hand and pumping it up and down. 'I really felt it to be necessary, the . . .'

'Oh, it was. Indeed it was, Miss Pillsworth,' I said, trying to get into my car. The night was warm and balmy but then

I realised that really, it was morning and I was tired and my mouth was dry. 'Two heads are better than one as they say. Oh dear . . .'

I was just about to drive off when she stuck a form through the window. It was to prove I'd made the visit, a proof for payment. I told her she could send it to me and I'd post it back. I ignored her protestations that really she'd prefer it done now, and before I could vent my irritation I drove off. She had been right to call me even though prematurely, but her lack of savvy in wanting me to sign a comparatively complicated form so early in the morning riled me. Kate Pillsworth riled me, period.

I meant to ask my secretary to remind me about Wendy Cotton, the girl Lee Kelly had asked me to see, but I forgot and had to rack my brains to remember who she was two days later when I was about to start my outpatients clinic at St Basil's. Oh yes, she didn't have an appointment, I told Sister Morgan, but I'd see her at the end of the clinic.

'Mrs Kane's here. Been waiting since one o'clock,' Morgan said.

I felt instant gloom. Mrs Kane's file was so large it was held together by tape. Coralie had attended almost every department of the hospital before being shunted to a psychiatrist some ten years ago. In spite of various acid notes by Doctor Ninian Gardener, my predecessor, to the effect that: 'This woman is a manipulative hysteric who seeks to get her way by lying, subterfuge and crude melodrama –' even he had been unable to shed Coralie. As soon as she was discharged she managed to be seen again by swallowing enough pills to gain admission to the hospital. Among the defeated letters from gastro-enterologists, cardiologists and surgeons and physicians, there were sheafs of correspondence from Social Services, the Gas Board, the Electricity Board and the Telephone Manager, plus considerable correspondence from the Housing Department. As well as being in constant war with the public services, Coralie had on several occasions been brought to court because of her debts, somehow managing to gain sympathy, in spite of her probation officer saying he was unable to help her because of her difficult personality.

Difficult personality just about summed it up. Coralie was egocentric, vain and extravagant. The State provided her with a maisonette and enough money to get by, if she managed it properly, but Coralie thought that life had been cruel to her and that she was owed not just a living, but a comfortable one. In spite of the many doctors she'd seen and their united opinion that she wasn't suffering from physical or mental disease, she chose to believe that there was something wrong with her that they were all missing and that they failed to appreciate her pathetic and lonely life. I had long given up arguing, especially since my suggestion that she should go to work was met with a storm of tears and the accusation that I had forgotten how pressure gave her 'blackouts'.

The obvious thing was to stop her coming to see me. Discharge her in fact, and stick to it ruthlessly. But then someone else would have to see her. I was confident that Coralie, with her malignant egotism, wasn't going to stay at home by herself when she'd been coming to hospital for years. And like GPs who saw their difficult patients merely as crosses to be born I had a weary notion that every doctor should take their share of unlikeable patients and Coralie was mine. Besides, if I didn't see her she'd bother her GP, poor Doctor Mary Langley, a saintly woman practitioner who was bravely carrying on her work in spite of bad rheumatoid arthritis.

'Good afternoon, doctor. Very hot isn't it? You'd think they'd have air conditioning in a place like this, wouldn't you? There's a woman out there turning a very nasty colour and I thought I was going to have one of my blackouts.'

Coralie tottered in on very high, black patent sandals. She always reminded me of a meringue, not the white kind but those pinky squashy ones. She was in her thirties and always looked the same. Her platinum hair was in the sleek Diana Dors style and her make-up was applied with the greatest care; pale blue eyes with correctly matching shadow and coral lips outlined with a skilled pencil. A barmaid, you'd have thought, or the wife of a carpet salesman. In spite of her sexy get-up, Coralie was at pains always to make clear that she was above 'that sort of thing'. Any man foolish enough to be taken in by the lushly curving bosom and smackable bottom, would find her sexually frigid I'd guess. She crossed her legs and smoothed back her hair with a small white hand, raspberry tipped and glittering with the large costume jewellery she affected.

'Well. And how are you, Coralie?' Ten minutes, that's all I'd give her. I was running late and there was Wendy Cotton to be seen.

'Up and down. Down mostly. The man opposite keeps playing the organ. He does it deliberately, you know. And the kids when they play . . . their language. Revolting. Downright disgusting it is.' The small pouting mouth was like a jam tart. 'And they vandalised the garage in front of the house, written up awful things I don't like to repeat . . .'

Then don't, I nearly said, but I knew that wouldn't put her off.

'Things like "Gertie is a slag" and "Sharon is a cunt". It's awful. I'm sick of reporting it. They take no notice.'

She should get out. Have a hobby. Do some voluntary work. I knew what I'd get and I got it.

'Work? With my nerves? You've got to be joking. I come over all queer if anyone looks at me. You know how I am . . .'

She pouted more than ever and went on in her most self-pitying tones that she was miserable, sad and lonely, without relatives, abandoned by the community. That stung me. I reminded her of her quarrel with at least two social workers, her complaints about the home help and her total refusal to go to a Community Day Centre, even though transport there and back would be provided.

'I know those sort of places. Make you spend all your time knitting and making baskets. I may be ill, Doctor, but I am not a fool.'

A handkerchief appeared and Coralie dabbed at her eyes which, probably to her annoyance because she was a very skilled actress, remained quite dry.

'Life can be very hard when you're on your own and have no one to stand up for you. When I go down to Doctor Langley she just gives me pills that upset me. I told her, I'm willing to *pay* just to get help but she took no notice. I feel I'm losing my reason. I'm going to crack-up completely, that's what's going to happen. Or I shall be found dead by the milkman...'

She began to sob loudly and I repeated what I'd told her so often, that the only way to forget her troubles was to get outside her house and involve herself with other people. To give the Community Day Centre a chance. Even if it bored her, she could at least try it.

'I haven't the strength to try. That's why I've come for help. Couldn't you give me some tablets to make me feel better, strong enough to get out...'

There it was. The same old search for the happy pills, the wonder drug that would make all effort unnecessary and provide not just rosy spectacles, but change life itself into a thing of joy where old age, pain and suffering were unknown. Coralie thought, as did so many other patients, that their NHS contributions should provide instant ease and that my attitude and refusal smacked of having my hand in the till.

As usual I seemed to have made her worse. She rose indignantly and stared at me furiously and reproachfully. For a minute I thought hurray, she's had enough, she's not going to come again, but I was wrong, of course. She shot her white appointment card at me and pouted peevishly when she saw what I'd written.

'The date seems so far away,' she said piteously. 'I may not be alive then.' But I steeled myself to stare impassively as she flounced out.

As the hours went by and the small room became like an oven, my hand grew cramped from writing and my voice hoarse from talking. The clinics seemed to get longer and longer, or was it my energy and tolerance getting in short supply? I was aware that my patience was definitely fraying and two of my patients looked at me solicitously and said I looked tired. I got really worried when I found myself prescribing a wrong dose. Tired doctors are dangerous ones. To cut medical corners was to court disaster and I wasn't just cutting, I was slicing.

Sister Morgan and her staff had gone home and the out-patients was silent and empty when I remembered Wendy Cotton. Maybe she'd gone. I couldn't blame her because it was nearly seven o'clock. But when I went out to look there she was, a thin girl in a creased dress sitting up very straight and watching the two middle-aged cleaners who were wielding polishers like bayonets as they shouted their comments on a television programme.

'In here, Mrs Cotton, sorry I kept you. I hope it's not put you out too much?'

'It's all right. There's nothing to do anyway till Ron, my husband, comes home.'

Oh yes. I skimmed the notes I'd made the first time I'd seen her. A year ago the problem had been her stammer.

'Mrs Kelly tells me you've done well. No stammer now.'

The girl stared around her blankly. Her small face was pinched with misery and her stringy hair hung in lifeless tendrils. She had a squint and her mouth hung open to reveal buck teeth. Even in health and with good make-up Wendy Cotton wouldn't have been good-looking, but now, depressed as she was, she was ugly. Since I'd seen her she'd got even thinner and her skimpy, yellow dress revealed a scraggy neck and stick-like arms.

'Oh, yes. I only stammer now and again. Very seldom really,'

Her voice wasn't local and then I remembered, she was a Cockney, born in Lambeth.

'What's the problem, Wendy? When I first saw you you told me you'd been married five years and had no children.' At the time I'd told her that there was still time. That she was only twenty-two and still very young. If, of course, the condition remained the same then she could go and see a specialist.

'That's what I done. I seen a specialist,' she said in a flat wooden voice. 'A gynaeco . . .'

'Gynaecologist?'

'That's right. He gave me a right going over. I had to go into hospital and have an examination and all. Had to have me tubes blown out and that.'

'And?'

The small face crumpled and from the way her voice wobbled I thought she was going to stammer again.

'And they found me womb wasn't normal. And me tubes are blocked. They told me I can't ever have a baby.'

Was she sure? They could do so much for infertility now.

'Course I'm sure. The specialist seen me and Ron, and he explained it all. Even made drawings. I can't ever have a baby . . .'

Well, there was always fostering. Or she could adopt?

'But it's not the same is it? Oh, it's not fair. It's not fair. It's not too much to ask to have a baby is it? I've never had nothing from life and that's for sure, but then I met Ron and he was so good to me that it was like there was some hope. Hope of things getting better. They couldn't get worse, could they?'

Ah, yes. Here it was. Wendy had had a very unhappy childhood. Her mother had dumped her in children's homes

43

and orphanages. Was that why she wouldn't consider fostering, I asked?

'Too right. I know what it's like, don't I? Personal experience. The times I used to wonder what me dad was like. I knew that me mother was a cow who only wanted me when it was too late and she had cancer. The nights I've spent thinking about what it was like to have a real mum and dad. The times I lay awake imagining a real home with real parents. Even bad ones would be better than none at all. And you know what kept me going? Thinking about how I'd have a baby of me own to love. I only had to remember how me mum treated me and do the opposite. I never ever thought I couldn't 'ave a kid. I didn't expect much of life. Never thought I'd find a bloke like Ron. But I always thought I'd be able to have a baby . . .'

She cried with loud chokes and hiccoughs, messily and convulsively like a child in bad pain. Any words would sound like platitudinous banality. I got up and walked over to her, putting an arm around her shuddering shoulders. I could feel the bones jutting out, sharp and angular.

'I can't stand it. I've tried to for Ron. He doesn't deserve to be tied to someone like me. Can't even give him a child. I dunno what I've done. I asked the specialist was it some badness in me blood? I know me mother slept around, she was never done talking about it when she had booze. And she used to say me dad came from a bad lot.'

I didn't think it was anything like that, I said, as Wendy tried to mop her face with the paper towel I handed her. Life had given her a very dirty deal I told her, and she was very depressed. What I'd like her to do would be to come into hospital and we would try and help her to feel better and maybe, when she was less depressed, she'd be able to think about the future. Maybe she could think of working in a day nursery? With her love of children she'd be a god-send.

'Not bloody likely,' she said between her sobs.

She wasn't nutty. There was nothing to be done. She'd only come here because Mrs Kelly had asked her to.

'And it's all right for her cause she's pregnant, isn't she?'

Oh dear, that must have been like sulphuric acid to poor Wendy's primitive ache.

'It was what kept me going. I felt as if there was something to live for looking forward to me baby.'

She began to weep again and I asked her what Ron felt. I was sure he loved her the same.

'So 'ee says. But he's a bloke, ain't he? Blokes don't feel the same. Anyway it's not doing right by 'im tethering 'imself to a barren old bag like me.'

I was very sure her husband didn't see her as a barren old bag I said. If she wouldn't come into hospital I'd write to her GP, Doctor Gillespie, and between us we'd do what we could to help her. I knew and liked Gillespie, who was a taciturn old Aberdonian whose heart was as broad as his accent.

'What can he do? What can you do? Nobody can help . . .' Wendy threw out her skinny arms like supplicating wands. There was something infinitely touching in her yearning gesture. She wrapped the thin arms around her bony body and bent forward in a movement so full of pain that I wanted desperately to help her, to be able to fill her empty soul and body with some sort of warmth.

'I know how hard it is, Wendy,' I said. 'Honestly, I know how you feel . . .'

The girl lunged back and bared yellow teeth at me. Her eyes were puffy and bloodshot and her shaggy hair fell over her ravaged face. 'Oh yes. You're all sorry for me. That's easy. But nobody can't do nuthin', can they? And all I want is what other women have. Just a baby. That's all. It's like being hungry all the time and I could put up with it before 'cause I thought it'd happen. I never thought it wouldn't. And I can't bear it . . .'

Her voice wavered and she was up and out before I could

say anything, let alone stop her. I tried to get Gillespie but he was in London the receptionist said. So it would have to wait till tomorrow. I picked up the powder compact that was near the phone. It must be Coralie's. The thought of her so plumply and self-righteously hard done by and the contrast with poor Wendy's true human misery depressed me. I was gathering myself up to go when the phone rang.

'Oh, Joyce. Glad I caught you. I tried to get you earlier but couldn't.'

Because it has been a hell of a day, I snapped, aware of my ratty tone. The flat voice of Coulter put the finish to a bad day. I started to tell him about the length of the clinic and the number of patients when he said, 'Listen. I'm ringing to say you've got an assistant. A Doctor Oliver Stafford.'

'That's quick work. How come?' I asked.

'Well. I met someone at Haxton where Stafford's been doing a locum which is now up. So he's free to come right away. He's married and will need accommodation, but that's no problem with the flat in the Priest's House being empty.'

That was fine, fine and dandy, I told Coulter. Had Stafford any experience in psychiatry?

'Plenty. I know the chap he's been working for and he speaks highly about him. Actually, I've got some good news myself. I've got a professorship in Maryland and will be taking it up as soon as I finish up here. Anyway, thought you'd like to know. I must pop off home now.'

Yes, good news, I thought driving home. Only question was, if Stafford was so good what was he doing taking locums in mid-career?

Chapter Four

I couldn't wait to phone Frankie but she'd gone out to a meeting Barney told me. He loathed the phone and it took him ages to answer. I could imagine him holding it the way he always did, half a foot from his ear, as if it was a dangerous incendiary. As he grumbled and groused about the terrible reception and the crackling noises, I told him that what I wanted Frankie for could wait and then I added that I was delighted to hear all was well with his chest.

'Well, you know what an alarmist Frankie is. Nothing's simple to you doctors, it is? I told Harper he was being too much of an old woman getting me X-rayed but he insisted. He'd complicate a rice pudding would Billy. I just went along for peace's sake.'

There was no greater alarmist than Barney, especially with his family history, but he was so pleased now it would be a shame to spoil his euphoria by mentioning that Harper was just being as careful as any good doctor. I was going to tell him that at last I was to have an assistant and then I thought to hell with it, Barney was already cursing and swearing about the bad line and I didn't want to tempt him into his favourite hobby of lambasting the telephonist, because there'd already been trouble about Barney's rudeness to a senior employee of the telephone company. Frankie said they'd have been cut off if it weren't for her being a doctor.

After supper I went over to the hospital library where there were reference books and medical directories. I found the entry on Oliver Stafford. He was in his thirties and had qualified in Wales after which there were residencies in very good teaching hospitals. He'd gained distinctions in his qualifying examinations and had done research at the Jackson Institute which was the foremost neurological centre in the country. Quite a hot shot was Stafford then. The question was why he wasn't settled in some permanent job by now. A bright young man like him should by now have achieved consultant-hood and not be taking locums. It didn't add up at all. And why was he taking junior jobs? Why not, with his track record, go for a senior appointment even at locum level? My brain raced over the possibilities. Maybe Stafford had poor health. If that was so then I hoped it was his physical health rather than his mental state, the statistics for mentally ill psychiatrists were significantly and shamefully high. Or maybe he had wife trouble. An unstable wife could pull any ambitious doctor down. I had to see Frankie. It was only half past nine maybe she'd soon be back from her meeting.

Frankie herself answered the door. She wore a smart cream dress and her hair was piled high. She looked blooming.

'Barney and me are just making a light supper of bacon and eggs. Join us?'

I said no, I'd eaten earlier, but I'd like some tea. As we went towards the kitchen I told her my news. Fantastic, great, she said and I wondered whether she'd taken in what I'd told her, especially as she rushed to the Aga where Barney was standing shaking the frying pan as if he were prospecting for gold. Frankie hovered irritably while Barney anointed his egg with oil.

'Swimming in grease, that's how he likes them, swimming in grease,' she tutted.

'And you like eggs like rubber bullets. Bollocks!' Barney roared as he slid his eggs on a plate and carefully placed the plate over a pan of hot water.

Frankie shot her egg in and began to slap oil on it while Barney shuddered and went over to the bottles on the dresser. Would I have a cocktail? he asked. He had a dated habit of serving cocktails and ever since he'd been entertained by some Americans in India he liked dry martinis. You had to watch him though because he was very heavy on the gin and his concoctions could be lethal. Frankie, who had now begun to fry bacon, said she'd have another.

I sipped my drink which tasted too like absolute alcohol for my liking and stared around the big old kitchen now full of the lovely smell of crisp bacon. Maybe I would have a bacon sandwich I told Frankie, while Barney yelled not to fry his to a cinder as he smacked down knives and forks on the huge deal table. The room had big windows from which billowed the pretty net curtains that Frankie had made from material bought at a Harrod's sale and the floor was covered with faded tiles. I looked out on to the garden where Willy, now that the day's heat had eased up a bit, was wearily sniffing around. The enormous old dresser, filling almost half one wall, was festooned with the many china jugs which were a hobby of Frankie's. There was a sewing machine on a marble table which had been brought back from a holiday in Florence, and a rich swathe of peacock silk fell silkily to the floor. Frankie as well as being a capable and experienced doctor was a dilettante with housework. She was an inspired, erratic cook and could have been an excellent dressmaker. If the mood took her she would decorate with demoniac industry and since I'd last been in the kitchen she'd painted all the cupboard and the walls with most professional expertise. Her mood was the thing though. If she got bored, then everything was shelved and she moved on to the next project. This drove Barney, who was obsessional, quite wild.

After downing his drink Barney went over to supervise his bacon and leaped backwards as a spurt of hot oil jetted towards his eye. 'Christ! Christ. I'm blinded! You had the heat too high, Frankie. Oh . . . Oh . . . Oh . . .' He hopped around the kitchen with his hand over his eye while Frankie

49

tried to get him to let her see it. 'Haven't you done enough damage? Do you want to finish me? I can't understand how a doctor can be so bloody clumsy. Keep away from me, for Christ's sake.'

Frankie stood unable to control her laughter while Barney bellowed in anguish.

'Wouldn't he drive you mad? He looks like a Cyclops,' she chuckled.

'I heard that, you cruel bitch!' Barney shrieked. 'Oh, my God . . . to be blinded as well as deafened. What a fate . . .'

I managed to get him to let me have a look at his eye while Frankie served the supper. The oil hadn't reached his eye, just burned the outer corner of the eyelid I said.

'Sure, I knew it wasn't much,' Frankie agreed. 'Let's eat.'

Barney revived and bent to eat his bacon and egg while Frankie, handing me a toasted bacon sandwich, asked about Oliver Stafford.

So she had taken in what I'd said. I had been beginning to feel a bit hurt at my old friend's apparent indifference to my news. In between bites of food I repeated what Coulter had told me and how I'd looked up Stafford in the medical directory.

'All very odd. Where's the catch?' Frankie mused.

That was exactly what I was wondering, I said, as Barney mopped up egg with a piece of crusty bread.

'What catch? What are you talking about?' Barney, even when he claimed his hearing was at it's worst, was adept at reading glances and interpreting expressions. 'Unless of course you don't want to tell me, Joyce. I know I must be like a stupid old fogey most of the time. It's an awful bore having to go over everything again so don't feel you have to.'

'Shut up and don't act the martyr,' Frankie snapped, as she cleared the table and began to make coffee.

I wasn't bored and it was no trouble, I said, and I told Barney what I'd told Frankie.

'I don't trust Coulter,' Frankie said. 'Do you know what I think? I think that he's taking Stafford to oblige a friend. A friend who in return for a favour would grant one to Coulter – like a professorship in America . . .'

'What would be obliging in taking Stafford?' I asked. 'You mean he could be trouble? Some scandal?'

'Something like that. This I'm sure of, Felix doesn't give one shit about you or the hospital, Joyce. But he wants out . . . to the States and he's using your need for help to do a favour . . '

I hadn't thought of that. I was overcome by the depressing possibilities raised by Frankie's theory. A doctor in trouble would really be worse than having to cope on my own. Wasn't that a bit melodramatic? I asked Frankie. Couldn't it just be bad health or a bad marriage marring a promising career?

'Could be. I hope so. It's just that Felix Coulter at the best of times hasn't even the cheese of human kindness, but Felix on the way out could be very dangerous.'

'Oh, for God's sake that's women all over,' Barney said, lighting a cheroot. His face shone with the glow of a good meal and the remains of back bacon grease.

Frankie began to dab at his mouth with a red table napkin and he ducked. 'Stop that, woman! You treat me like a moronic child at times. Frustrated maternal instinct and I can't stand women being obviously maternal. I say you should give this young fellow a chance and not down him before he starts. I'll bet it's wife trouble. Nothing like a woman for ruining a promising career. I had one CO who reckoned he could sniff out a wife who'd cause trouble in a station in two minutes. He was always right. Always. What I say, Joyce, is give the lad a chance . . .'

I didn't like the idea that I was going to down Oliver Stafford before I'd even seen him, so I said that maybe Frankie and I were steeped in the cynicism of years spent in the medical world.

'We're realists, not cynics,' Frankie said, pouring more coffee.

Barney threw some bacon bone over his shoulder at Willy, who had reappeared and was snuffling at his master's legs. Barney leaned over and patted the old dog, saying he thought there must be something of Henry the Eighth in him because he loved to have a dog to toss a bone to.

Oh yes, he shared more than that taste with Henry, Frankie said, as she sliced into a fruit flan.

Then Barney read us a lecture about prejudging Stafford. Give the man a chance, see how he shapes up. After all, the post wasn't permanent, only a locum.

Changing the subject, I told Frankie about Wendy Cooper and that reminded her of another patient of mine, a girl called Sheena Boden. Sheena had been stricken down with a florid and acute attack of schizophrenia for which she'd had treatment in Barrington Hall. She was found to have diabetes as well, as if fate hadn't been unkind enough to her. However, she had made a very good recovery in spite of us all thinking that she wouldn't make it, that she'd gone too far along the dark road into the worst form of madness. She was helped by her love for her three-year-old daughter, Melinda. The idea that she had a reason for living, that her child was depending on her, had been more therapeutic than any drug, I was sure of that.

Frankie and Barney had taken the mother and child in for a few weeks after discharge from hospital. They had been kind and warm to the girl and so loving to the child that Sheena had been afraid, she told me, that Melinda would be spoiled rotten. Now Sheena was stabilised on a new drug which kept her sane and had come to terms with her diabetes after a tussle with the bureaucracy of Social Services who were initially, and perhaps rightly, a bit worried that Sheena wouldn't be able to cope, so had placed the child in a foster home. She was coping magnificently now. A small but centrally placed maisonette was given to her and, what with the odd visit from a social worker and the district nurse, Sheena was raising her child by herself and gaining confidence all the time.

'Sheena was doing fine last time I called to see her,' I said. 'Which reminds me, I must visit her again soon. She's got an excellent social worker, Patsy Godwin, keeping an eye on her.'

Barney suddenly announced that he was going for a walk and Willy came to life with a small panic of joy.

'Talking of social workers, have you come across one called Kate Pillsworth?' I asked.

'Don't think so. What's she like?'

'Amazonian. With a mop of rusty curls and a very earnest manner.'

'Say no more. Yes, I do know her. She's a menace. She upset poor old Doctor Eustace because she kept telling a patient that she should insist on this and that test from him.'

'Of course, she's young. And full of principles and ideals. I give her full marks for a grating manner, but equally full ones for caring. She reminds me of a missionary heroine in ways. But she's inexperienced. She'll learn I suppose.'

'Pity she has to cut her wisdom teeth on us,' Frankie said and, as she reheated the coffee, I told her about Mr Dippy.

'That's priceless. Fancy giving a strict Muslim a pork chop. I must tell Barney. He'll enjoy that.'

When Barney came back over an hour later it was to find us still chatting about patients and he waved his stick impatiently. 'I don't know what you two will do when you retire. We had a good rule in the army. Positively no shop in the mess.'

'Listen. You must hear about this poor little Mr Dippy . . .'

Frankie was about to tell him when Barney began to cough. The spasm was so bad that he had to lean over the kitchen table, his whole body racked with the convulsive heaving. I didn't like the blue-white pallor of his face when at last the spasms lessened, and I could see by Frankie's anxious face that she didn't either.

'Here. Drink this.' She poured some water and handed him a glass. His hands were shaking and some of the water spilled, but he managed to retain some gulps and Frankie said solicitously that he should go up to try to rest, preferably in bed.

'What kind of bloody advice is that, Frankie? You know I hate bed and you know how I'm cursed with insomnia. For years I've been trying to get some doctor to take an interest and try to find me some medicine that will help me sleep. I must have swallowed a crumb the wrong way or something. I'll go and have a snifter of brandy.' He marched out rather unsteadily, followed by Willy.

'He's not well. I hope the X-ray's all right.'

Frankie looked so worried that I reminded her of Barney's iron constitution and that he smoked too much. Nothing more than a smoker's cough I added, though I didn't like the coughing spells either.

'Nobody's going to stop him having his cheroots. Not me, nor Harper, nor God Almighty Himself. It's the family history . . .'

'Yes,' I agreed. No use producing more anodynes to fear. We both had seen too many patients die after a chest cancer, lung cancer, which had started, in most cases insidiously, by a cough put down to cigarettes.

The price of a medical education is that you know the options and the lack of them. Again I tried to reassure Frankie. Barney did everything extravagantly I reminded her, his insomnia was not the woe he described it, especially since he invariably slept in the afternoon. And what about the way he enjoyed his food in spite of his fixed belief that he ate hardly enough to keep a fly alive? He had a cough, but Harper hadn't found anything and I was sure the X-ray would be clear. When was he having it?

'Day after tomorrow. I'd better see how he is.'

I would have to go I said, and on the way home I remembered that I was to try and talk to Doctor Gillespie about Wendy Cotton. And call to see Sheena Boden.

It could be hell trying to get a busy GP of a morning but I was in luck and got Ian Gillespie first time.

'I saw a patient of yours, Wendy Cotton, yesterday. She's terribly distressed about not being able to have a child. Really so disturbed that I wanted to admit her and try to do something for her depression.'

'Aye. She's a sad lass. The ones who don't want kids are often over-fertile and yet there's that poor girl can't have any. She had a deprived childhood and got tuberculosis of her pelvis; the inflammation was so bad that it's scarred all the reproductive organs beyond repair. Just one of those awfully sad cases where one can't do anything.'

'I think we might be able to help support her till she comes to some kind of terms with herself,' I said. 'I can't help her to have a child, but I may be able to get her to the stage where she can think about adoption. But at the moment she's refusing all help and is just in complete despair. I was wondering whether you'd be able to persuade her to come to the clinic again?'

'I'll try to have a talk with her. Matter of fact I have a call to do near Wendy. If she agrees to come and see you again, when shall I tell her?'

'I'll see her any time at the clinic at St Basil's. No appointment necessary.'

That was that. Probably Wendy wouldn't turn up. But I thought of her stark misery and the agonised supplication of her arms, and I hoped she would.

I was lucky with Sheena, because she had just come in from a walk in the park with Melinda, who was now asleep on the divan. She was a pretty little girl with long, straight flaxen hair and Sheena's smutty eyes.

'Would you like some coffee, Doctor Delaney?'

Sheena was wearing blue denims and a white T-shirt. With her honey-coloured hair pinned back with a red ribbon and her biscuity tan, she was like any attractive young girl. Hard to imagine the desperate girl with the delusions and hallucinations that made her appear like a demented monkey. There had been so many days when she had crouched in a side room, spitting when anyone came near her and gibbering wildly to the gallery of her inner demons. Impossible to imagine that that witch-like girl bore any resemblance to the happy kid who was pouring coffee into a red mug.

'And you must try these, I made them myself.'

I took one of the oatmeal cookies and looked around the large, sunny flat. There wasn't much furniture to be sure, but Sheena was artistic and the paintings and posters on the white-washed walls made a brave show. The floor had been sanded and varnished and Sheena said that the social worker might be able to get her a carpet. I sat down on a large settee which Sheena had covered with brown velvet that she'd got at a sale.

'Have another cookie.'

As I took another I asked her how she was getting on, although maybe there was no need to ask that. She looked so well and Melinda was obviously thriving.

'She's fine.' Sheena bent over the sleeping child. The small limbs were as slack and relaxed as only a child's can be and Sheena removed a bit of fluff from her daughter's hair. Madonna in Jeans I thought, looking at the mother and daughter. 'I feel marvellous,' Sheena moved away from Melinda and stretched her brown arms upwards. 'I love my flat. And people are so kind. Some students from the university heard about me and they come twice a week and chat. Sometimes we go to the pub for a drink and this weather they've been taking Mel and myself out for a drive. Everything's super, Doctor . . .'

My pleasure in seeing Sheena and her child happy and settled made up a little for my worry about Wendy Cotton. Sheena thanked me at the door for all I'd done. She was ever so grateful, she didn't know how to thank me.

'All I did, Sheena,' I said, 'was to help you grit your teeth. My reward is seeing you so well.'

It was still glorious weather. The prophets had been right in their forecasts and there was even talk of a drought. I decided to take some time off and went shopping in Yorkely, after which I went for a walk in the park. I stayed there till the rush of traffic was over and then I drove home. Funny, I thought when I reached the Priest's House again, curtains in the lower flat. And the downstairs door into the bottom flat was open. I couldn't resist having a peep inside. A dark haired young woman was bent over a packing case.

'Are you Mrs Stafford?' I asked and she smiled and came towards me. She was very pretty with a sort of marble perfection which came alive, broke up, when she smiled. Her eyes were hazel with very dark lashes framing them. 'I'm Doctor Delaney. I live in the top flat.'

'I'm pleased to meet you. I'm expecting Oliver any minute. He went into town for some bulbs.'

Very Welsh cadence to the voice.

'Would you like some tea? Or any sort of help? I didn't know you were coming today.' Trust Felix not to bother telling me the Staffords had arrived.

'Oh, no. Not at all. It won't take us long. We're used to packing and unpacking.'

Did I detect anything in the way she said that? A hint of longing for a more settled life?

'Have you a family, Mrs Stafford? Or . . .'

'No. Just the two of us. Would you like me to make you some tea? It won't take long.'

'No thanks, no, really,' I said. 'Do let me know if there's anything I can do. Anything you're not sure of. I expect your husband will want to give you a hand, so I won't expect him at the hospital for a day or two.'

'We're used to moves,' she said. 'It shouldn't take us long to settle in. It's lovely to have such a spacious flat. Our last one was tiny. And the garden is a bonus.'

'Charlie, the gardner, is dedicated,' I said. 'Yes, it's a fine, solid old house. I'm glad to have people underneath.'

'Just as long as we don't disturb you, Doctor Delaney,' Olwyn said.

'Call me Joyce. And do tell your husband he doesn't have to turn up for work right away.'

'I don't think I'll be able to stop him,' Olwyn said, and when a fat black cat appeared and began to rub himself against her legs she smiled and added, 'This is our cat, Satan. I hope you don't mind?'

'You having a cat? It'll help to keep the mice down.'

Later, over my supper, I could hear the noise of furniture being moved around and there were a few thuds and bumps and doors banging. But as I'd told Olwyn, it was nice to feel that I wasn't alone. It was also nice to have an assistant. Maybe I'd be able to do some of the things I'd put on the long finger. I might be able to manage two holidays instead of one. It looked as if Felix Coulter, in spite of my cynical reservations, had done me a good turn. He had personal motivation, I was sure of that; his American connection had surely been forged in Haxton, but as Barney would say, 'What the hell.'

Chapter Five

I looked out hopefully for Wendy Cotton at my next clinic at St Basil's but she wasn't there. Not that I thought she'd come even though Gillespie could be very persuasive. While I was half expecting to see Stafford, there was no sign of him, despite my having heard them both moving around in the flat below me. The walls of the old house were substantial and the building was sound structurally, so there was good insulation and I couldn't hear voices. The clinic was quite small and I finished in good time. At least I thought I'd finished, when I heard an apologetic cough and a neatly dressed man appeared.

'Harold Martin's the name, Miss . . . I mean, Doctor . . .'

He wasn't on my list. Sister Morgan must have slipped up and forgotten to put the name in. Doctor Melling, the GP, wasn't too forthcoming either. Mr Martin was depressed and low-spirited, unable to mix with people.

'Very good of you to see me, Doctor.' Martin wore a dark suit with a stiff-collared shirt and a red tie neatly secured with a gold tie-pin. His voice was meek and he smoothed back some strands of grey hair over his balding head.

'Well now, Mr Martin, what can I do for you?'

'You mean what is the matter with me?'

'That's it. Yes.'

'Well. I live on my own, I have a small flat actually, and I get rather lonely.'

'What about your job? People often find they make friends at work.'

'That would be difficult with my job. You see, I'm a night-watchman.'

Half an hour later I'd decided that what Mr Martin

needed was a wife, and that he'd be better joining a social club or something of that sort. There was nothing at all obviously psychiatric the matter with him and I was beginning to think that he was just a pleasant, ageing man who was on his own too much. Had he never thought of marrying?

'Oh, yes. I was married for twenty years.'

'Was?'

'My wife is dead.'

Sad, I said, wondering whether I should even ask him what his wife died of.

He looked so tragic sitting looking down at his hands which were folded on his lap. So melancholy the way his voice faltered as he said, 'Yes. Lily is dead.'

What did she die of? I asked him.

He cleared his throat. 'I murdered her.'

I wondered had I heard him right or was he becoming deluded? Perhaps this was some sick fantasy of a disordered mind?

'I shot her. Twenty times. Proper mess she was.' The calm, measured tones and the way he stared impassively at me made it all the more bizarre. 'She was always unfaithful to me. All the time I was away during the war. And after. I stood for most of it because I never thought of myself as exciting or able to give her the good times she wanted. But when Lily started going out with a pig called Jimmy Nester I couldn't take it. He was an animal . . .'

For a moment something dark and nasty showed in the mild, pasty coloured face and watery brown eyes.

'She taunted me one day. All tarted up she was, ready for meeting Nester and she told me she was sick of the sight of me and wanted to go away with Nester. She said I wasn't half the man he was. So I killed her.'

No remorse, no drama, just the flat facts, so starkly delivered that it made it the more horrific. Eyes steady and holding my gaze unblinkingly, he continued:

'I'm a fair shot. So they said in the army and I kept in practice.'

What had happened after the shooting? Had he gone to prison? I asked.

'I got twenty years. Done ten in Winston Green but the Parole Board let me out when I done ten because of good behaviour.'

That figured. I could imagine him ingratiating himself with the screws and getting a cushy number in the prison hospital. All the same, even this emotionless character must have suffered deeply in the harsh atmosphere of prison. There was bound to be psychological scarring and areas of bitterness in Martin, leaving him with a deep grudge against society. As I tendered my sympathy and condolences he smiled thinly.

'I think you got it wrong, Doctor. I liked being in prison. You had no worries and you had company and companionship. I wish I was back.'

It transpired that Martin had a good job as a watchman with a small flat near the job. But he was lonely and isolated with only his four walls. He wasn't a drinking man, he told me primly, and found socializing impossible. Always shy and diffident he'd become desperately nervy in company, fearing that he'd drop something about prison or that people would find out about it and shun him. He was terrified of rebuff but anxious to make human contact, especially, as he said, 'Amongst the opposite sex.'

He wasn't mentally ill and looked, in his dark suit and a mac folded over his arm, ultra respectable. I'd send him someone from Social Services who would suggest some social clubs he could join. He smiled, thanked me for my time and walked quietly out.

I called at Frankie's on the way home. She and Barney were relaxing in the front room. Barney, with Willy under the chair, was reading Trollope and Frankie was putting the finishing touches to a kaftan made from the exotic peacock coloured silk. I told her all about meeting Olwyn Stafford.

'She sounds all right. Nothing obviously wrong. Quite a suet pudding in fact,' she said, biting thread with her strong teeth.

'Not in appearance,' I said. 'In fact, she's almost too beautiful, except when she smiles. Lovely pale skin and the sort of profile that would go well on a medallion. And slanted eyes. Very Welsh.'

'The Welsh are a devious lot,' Barney barked suddenly. He had appeared to be deep in Barchester, but then he adored a bit of gossip and seldom missed hearing any despite his deafness. 'We had a medical officer from Abergavenny once and he cheated at bridge. And I've always heard that they're dirty rugger players.'

'It's a good job the racial discrimination people don't get a load of you,' Frankie said, snapping thread again. She held out the finished garment and stared at it, satisfied.

'Lot of rot talked about race. They go banging on about equal rights for the coloured. When I spent two years in South Africa I heard on all sides that the Bantu were stupid buggers. What's the good of trying to educate the un-educable? Someone told me the Bantu had abnormally thick skull bones.'

'Listen to him,' Frankie said drawing the curtains. 'Fascism unconfined.'

Trollope was forgotten as Barney launched into his theme, 'It's a question of culture, not colour,' Barney said. 'Take the Indians. They're a rice-eating culture, right? And you won't change that for a long time. What the hell does an Indian doctor know about the mores of a housewife in Yorkely? And yet they're still letting Indians into the country. It's like the importation of cheap Japanese goods.'

'We'll have Kipling next,' Frankie said, 'with a touch of Powell for good measure.'

I could see the danger of a battle, so I cut in and asked

about Barney's X-ray. He'd had it, Frankie said, and singed the radiographers ears with his language.

'What's that you're saying?' Barney twiddled with his hearing aid.

'I was telling Joyce how you behaved while you were having your X-ray. The air was dark navy blue.'

'Rubbish. I felt bloody ridiculous in that stupid little robe they gave me to wear, having to hold my breath lying trussed like a fowl for roasting. All that bloody machinery. You doctors do this to terrify people to death.'

I wished I hadn't mentioned the X-ray, especially when Frankie said they hadn't had the result yet because the radiologist was ill and couldn't read the plates till tomorrow.

'This cursed thing's on the blink again.' Barney scrabbled at his hearing aid and wrenched it from his ear. He was red and cross-looking and ranted about the iniquitous state of affairs when businessmen made money out of foisting useless hearing aids on the infirm.

'It's because you don't clean the machine,' Frankie said.

Barney reared up asking how she'd like to have to spend her time scraping at a hearing aid like picking invisible winkles? It was no good, he continued, querulous and irascible.

On the way out, Frankie told me that she'd bet anything he was secretly worried about his X-ray.

It would be all right, I assured her. But would she phone me when it came through?

'It'll probably show two lungs fibrosed with nicotine,' Frankie said.

The weather broke next day and there was a sudden and violent storm during the night, bringing sheets of rain which cooled and freshened the parched air. The deluge wouldn't keep patients away even if they had to charter their own arks.

'I'm in a bit of a tiz today,' Morgan panted, explaining that all the Senior House Officers had been changed around and she didn't know where she was with trying to steer all the strange young doctors so that they knew where they were and what they should be doing. Morgan's know-how and expertise at out-patient work made her the scourge of housemen, especially those she called the 'uppity ones'. Morgan had favourites and showed it.

The first patient to arrive, glowing and glamorous in pink plastic and cellophane overboots was Coralie Kane. She teetered in and removed her overboots to reveal dainty, black suede sandals. She felt she was dying. Didn't know how she'd got through the weekend she grumbled, holding her middle as she sank on to the chair. The GP hadn't been on and when she phoned she couldn't make out what the answering phone was saying, so she'd called the police and they'd managed to get her one of the relief doctors who hadn't been at all helpful.

'He wore sort of jeans and he had long hair. Didn't know what to make of me. He asked me all sorts of questions and then said I'd better come and see you.'

That was the Emergency Service for you I thought. What exactly was she complaining of? I asked Coralie as she fluffed at her silvery hair. She pulled down her pouting bee-stung mouth and then began to prod at her chest and stomach.

'I get this darting pain in my shoulders then it goes down to me tummy . . .' She spread her silver tipped hand in the general direction of her plump abdomen. 'And I feel me heart thundering like. I sometimes think it's going to burst. Have you ever had a patient whose heart burst?'

Before giving me time to answer she continued the description of her visitations.

'Me stomach feels bloated and I come over all hot and cold . . .'

Perhaps it was the advent of the menopause I said, rather unkindly.

'Doctor . . . and me only in my early thirties?' she said reproachfully.

She'd been fully investigated physically, I told her, and these 'turns' were nothing more than anxiety about herself causing her heart to beat rapidly. She then swallowed more air than usual and this caused her heavy, bloated feeling. Everything was made worse by the fact that she didn't mix with people and had no friends.

'Friends? People don't want you when you have no money. Women are especially nasty. They think you're after their men, though why they should think that I have no idea.'

I bit back the opinion that maybe if she dressed less like an available tart other women might trust her more.

She rummaged in her black patent bag for the handkerchief which was one of her props. She thought that being a woman I'd understand, she went on. She'd been getting obscene phone calls she said.

That made a change from reading graffiti I was going to add. But instead I asked her why she didn't tell the police.

'They don't want to know,' she answered crossly. 'Just don't want to know. One of them arrived in a Panda after I'd reported the calls and he looked at me in ever such a peculiar way and pressed my hand on the way out. I was going to report him for familiarity. I think I know who's behind the calls. It's a woman on the estate, a rat-bag whose husband left her. I was thinking, Doctor, what about me coming into hospital for a rest? I could come into Flower Ward. A lady outside was telling me it helped her.'

No, no, and no, I told her. I always resisted this request, which came up regularly. If Coralie came into hospital she'd get firmly dug in, and the admission would convince her that she was really ill. Plus the fact that it wouldn't be fair to subject the nursing staff to the wiles of a designing woman like Coralie.

There was a knock on the door and a man came in. I had

an impression of raven black hair, sallow skin and dark eyes which had a burning intensity. He would be handsome if it weren't for the worn black suit and the pallor of his skin.

'Oliver Stafford,' he said.

I shook hands with him and asked Coralie to wait outside.

'Certainly,' she said, fluttering her eyelashes at Stafford. 'I don't mind at all. But I do have some other things to tell a doctor . . . I don't mind which doctor.'

I wasn't surprised at Coralie's ogle but Stafford seemed, if not returning Coralie's glance, to be looking at her with pleasure.

I had an idea. When Coralie had gone out I asked Stafford if he had formally started work. Yes, he said, and he hoped that I'd give him something to do.

'Well. I hesitate to inflict Coralie Kane on you.'

'The pretty girl who just went out?' he asked.

Funny, I'd never thought of Coralie as a 'pretty girl'; depended on your taste I supposed. I gave him a run down on the Kane psyche. I hoped that he might even be able to discharge her, though I doubted it. Had he been in psychiatry long? After I'd asked the question I felt foolish because, of course, when I'd looked up his entry in the medical directory there had been the record of his work in psychiatric hospitals. And there had been Haxton, of course. He gave me a run down on his previous jobs in an easy, almost chatty way. His voice was deep and more Welsh than his wife's. Then he suddenly said, looking at me, 'But of course you'll have already looked me up, won't you?'

Of course, I said, trying to sound natural and easy. I gave him a few openings to find out why he'd left Haxton so quickly, but I got nowhere. Either he was a skilled parryer or plain didn't want to tell me. Probably the latter I thought, and asked whether his wife had settled in.

'Oh, yes. Olwyn's fine. She's got herself a job in a law firm in Yorkely.'

My, my, that was quick work, I thought. The Staffords were certainly sharp and speedy operators. Yet, as I talked to Stafford, I wasn't conscious of his being slippery. He sounded pleasant, sensible and with a great enthusiasm.

'Would you mind giving me a run down on what you would like me to do work-wise, Doctor Delaney? I'd like to start as soon as possible.'

That was O.K. by me I said. I'd been without an assistant for so long it would be grand to have help. Then I outlined his work. Stafford had really amazing eyes, deep set and glowing when he got animated, he was now using his hands like a Latin to emphasise points.

'How many Community Nurses have you got here? They've just appointed two at Haxton.'

We had four I told him, and they were really excellent at checking that discharged patients kept up their treatment, and kept an eye on the patients who lived on their own or had bad home surroundings.

'Listen,' I said. 'I'll take you around my "patch" after the clinic if you like.'

Fine, he said, getting up and shaking ash from his knee. And he would see Coralie for me.

After he'd gone I felt a bit of a heel off-loading Mrs Kane on a willing victim like Stafford. But he was experienced enough to spot the sort of woman she was and cope with her machinations and manipulations. You never know, he might manage to discharge her.

He tapped at my door an hour or so later and I said 'How did you make out with Coralie Kane? She's a shocker isn't she?'

'Do you think so?'

'Don't *you*?' I asked in surprise.

Well, she had a difficult personality in some ways, he said, paranoid and aggressive. But he felt that perhaps he should get to know her better and then assess just what he could do to help. He was very interested in psychotherapy and had done two years of training for it at the Park Clinic in London.

Impressive. The Park Clinic was very prestigious and only took on very good doctors; it was in the position of calling the tune and had many applicants.

Coralie had asked what psychotherapy meant and he'd explained that what it really meant was that the client and the therapist 'talked things out' over a period, and thus self-knowledge developed, helping the adjustment to life and relationships. Mrs Kane had never had a real relationship with anyone because her parents had been elderly and hadn't wanted a child anyway, and her husband had been an invalid who wanted a housekeeper not a wife. Yes, Mrs Kane seemed keen all right and well motivated to attend for regular sessions.

I judged it wise to try to warn him about Coralie and her shallow, hysterical nature but he simply smiled politely. To hell with it, I thought, maybe Coralie *can* benefit by his treatment and I've been remiss in diagnosing her as a selfish nuisance and an emotional leech. New Doctor Syndrome? Well, maybe. It was a fact that a strange doctor often saw things a patient's normal practitioner might have missed. He, a graduate of the Park Clinic, must know his psychotherapeutic onions.

'Let's go to Barrington,' I said. 'Do you have a car?'

'Afraid not. I use a bike which I motorised myself. Olwyn calls it my put-put bike.'

In that case, since he hadn't come on his bike, I'd give him a lift. On the way back Oliver chatted to me in an easy and relaxed fashion. He didn't boast, didn't indulge in any clinical name-dropping, but I knew that he was experienced and knowledgeable by what he said. Of course, there were plenty of doctors who were bursting with theory and blindingly brilliant in their cerebral ability. Maybe Oliver didn't come across at the bed-side, lacked the rapport with a patient which made medicine an art as well as a craft. I must try to squeeze some information from Coulter, although I hadn't seen him for days and his secretary said she thought he had left the hospital and was busy at home making last-minute arrangements.

I had an example of Oliver's clinical nous after we'd tramped around all my wards and ended up on Flower Ward where Sister Gabriel, a pretty West Indian, was having trouble with one of her patients. Nancy Gabriel was quiet, a bit reserved and lacking the ebulliance which I'd come to expect with West Indians. You had to know her for a long time before she relaxed with you and there was a hint of sadness in her eyes, as if somewhere along the line she'd been hurt. She was reticent about her past but her patients loved her and now, after working with her for two years I liked her and found that behind the soft voice and the rather reserved manner, Nancy Gabriel had quite a sense of humour.

Oliver Stafford talked easily to her without appearing to hammer her with questions. As he talked he leaned back in his chair, long limbs draped and those strange, smouldering eyes registered his complete immersion in what the other person was saying. I could tell that Sister Gabriel liked him. He certainly seemed to have a gift for establishing rapport with women.

'Any immediate problems, Sister?' I asked when we'd finished tea.

'Nothing that can't wait till tomorrow. Doreen Winters came back to us, by the way.'

'Is she pregnant? I mean, did she see Doctor Gill?' Gill was one of the obstetricians at St Basil's.

'She did and she isn't. I mean she saw Doctor Gill and he told her she's not pregnant.'

'Then how does he explain the gain in weight? And her periods stopping?'

And there was Doreen's own intelligence. She said that the pattern for her last two children had been the same.

Periods ceased but there was still a slight 'show' of blood every month and she had a sudden and marked enlargement of her abdomen. She had already been told she wasn't pregnant by her GP and this was the last straw. Mixed up and anxious as she was, the more than a hint that she was imagining things had blown her wide open.

Also, they weren't very nice to her at St Basil's where they implied that because she was in Barrington she must be a pseudocoyesis or phantom pregnancy. She was in bed weeping and upset about being made to feel potty, Gabriel went on. I said that no matter what Gill said I thought Doreen was pregnant. Who better than a mother of four to know the pattern of her pregnancies and there *was* the fact that her protuberant abdomen looked distinctly pear-shaped and pregnant?

'Nurse Jones, who went down with her, said Doctor Gill was very abrupt and impatient. Jones says she heard he was going to send you a sarcastic letter, Doctor Delaney.'

I was used to that, I said. General hospitals still treated psychiatric patients like time wasting nuisances at times.

We went into the dormitory and there was poor Doreen lying on a bed sobbing. She was a small, mousy girl with enormous frightened eyes. Damn, she had improved so much we were thinking of discharge and now this. Even if she wasn't having a child, why didn't Gill exercise more tact? And when I slipped her nightie up to reveal the abdomen swelling tight and drum-like I felt the foetus. I was sure of it. But I didn't have anything to hear the foetal heart with; maddening because I was convinced, leaning right over the girl's tummy, that I could hear the unmistakable thrumming of the fast intra-uterine beat.

Oliver whipped out the small instrument used to check the heart of a baby in the womb. He always carried one, he said, patting his inner jacket where the percussion hammer, stethoscope and opthalmoscope nestled. He murmured gentle encouragement to Doreen who was shivering with cold and agitation and then, after listening at different parts of the tight, white abdomen, he said quietly, 'It's here. Just where I'm listening. Unmistakable.'

So it was, I found out when he moved back to let me listen. I could hear, over the spot on the lower right part of the girl's abdomen, the baby's galloping heart beating at quite a different rhythm to Doreen's own.

'You're going to be a mother again, dear,' Oliver smiled at the patient who sighed.

'Thank God. We didn't want another but we'll manage. I'm sorry for carrying on, Doctor, but Doctor Gill was so nasty to me when he told me I wasn't pregnant that I felt desperate and thought I was going potty.'

'It happens to all doctors; we make mistakes sometimes,' I said to Oliver on the way home, 'So it doesn't behove Gill to be Smart Alecy. I'll send him a snooty letter.'

When we got to the Priest's House Oliver asked me in for coffee. I didn't really want any but thought it would be churlish to refuse. Olwyn, who had been sitting in a rocker stroking Satan, jumped up and seemed delighted to see us. She looked fresh as paint in a red skirt and white blouse, young and delicately pretty enough to always look well, or else I'd never come across her on an 'off day'. Watching the Staffords together as they chatted happily over the coffee making, I couldn't imagine them being other than harmonious. Unless they were consummate actors, but even then could they sustain an act. Oh well, as Frankie had said, time would reveal any chinks and flaws.

I sipped at the mug of coffee Olwyn handed me. The kitchen was old and nothing could be done about the flagged floor and the dingy ceiling but the old gas stove, almost a collector's item, seemed to have been put to good use because there were two fresh loaves cooling. Olwyn followed my glance.

'We hate the shop bread so we take it in turns to bake our own.'

'We?'

'Oliver, too. He can sew better than me and he's a very good knitter.'

A man of many talents, Stafford, I thought. Obviously thoroughly domesticated.

'Only thing I can't get him to do is to take an interest in his clothes. He goes out like a tramp sometimes. But on the whole he's a workaholic.'

'Don't be so daft, Ol. You make me sound like a monster.'

They looked at each other with the almost secret and living complicity you get in a sound relationship.

I asked Olwyn how her job was going and where she worked.

'Oh . . . it's a solicitor's office. Quite interesting. There's three partners and they're all very nice to me. In fact everyone has been so kind and helpful I think we're going to be very happy in Yorkely.'

I'd loved to have asked her how she got the job, got fixed up so very quickly, but instead I said, 'And I'm delighted to have such an experienced assistant.'

Later, when I got back to my own flat I phoned Frankie. How was the X-ray?

'That's the thing. The radiographer was inexperienced and the plates weren't too clear. But they think all is well. I'm not saying anything to Barney and have sworn Harper to secrecy.'

'Aren't they going to re-X-ray?'

'Barney wouldn't hear of it. I only got him to go in the first place by cashing in on his being a bit rattled. If I told him the X-rays were bungled he'd only get more paranoid about doctors and hospitals. Best leave well alone for the time being. What's your news? Has Stafford arrived?'

Yes, I said, and told her about the events of the day and

how I was just up from the Staffords' who seemed a loving and united couple.

'All very odd,' Frankie said. 'Curiouser and curiouser. I mean his coming here just like that with no notice and that.'

That could be planned. It made a certain sense to take locums while you were sniffing around for a permanent job.

'I suppose so,' Frankie said. 'Haven't you leaned on Felix to see if you can get any more information?'

That was the thing, I said, I hadn't been able to track down Coulter but I intended to try to do so tomorrow.

'Of course, when I thought old Felix might be a homo I would have said that he'd been loitering with intent at some lav' in London and found Stafford, or else gone to the Hammersmith Palais and picked him up there.'

For God's sake! I had to laugh. Never, I told Frankie, had there been such a ridiculous and unlikely reason thought up for engaging a locum.

'Yeah. Maybe it's a bit too melodramatic.' Frankie yawned. 'All, as they say, will be revealed.'

Chapter Six

I tracked Felix down next day, although he wasn't in the least forthcoming about Stafford when I did run him to earth. Indeed, I began to think that Frankie's dramatic theory of 'favours' might have some substance.

'I don't know much about Doctor Stafford,' Coulter said vaguely. 'Just that Haxton's say he was a good worker and very experienced in psychiatry. Always pleasant and obliging, too.'

That was precisely it, I said, Stafford was such an academic high-flyer that it was odd that he hadn't got promotion. Young men, the bright ones anyway, just didn't traipse around the country doing locums.

'People have all sorts of reasons for their actions,' Coulter said. 'You as a psychiatrist should know that.'

Yes, but as a psychiatrist I was also interested in motives, I said, and Coulter smiled his blandest smile.

'You're getting institutionalised, Joyce, seeing everybody as case histories. You've got what you asked for, a good assistant who can speak English.'

He had me there. I was always saying that to practise psychiatry with any small success you need to speak English and Coulter himself had ticked me off one day and called me a racist.

'Touché, Felix,' I said.

He began to arrange papers in his brief-case with almost obsessional care. He had to go, he said. So much to do, because the Area Health Authorities had agreed to waive their six months' notice requirement for him and he was flying to America next week and the family were following at the end of the month.

'Exit Felix then,' said my colleague Toby Manners in the cafeteria at lunch. 'We must see that the advertisement for his replacement goes into the journals pronto. How is your new assistant doing? I hear on the grapevine that he's pretty good.'

Very good, I said. I didn't think I'd have much to teach him. It was funny though that Stafford hadn't gone higher. And suspicious that Coulter had been so quick to oblige me. I told Manners about Frankie's observations.

'Trust Frances to sus it out,' he commented. 'Still, maybe we're wrong to be so full of doubts. I should relax and enjoy it if I were you. I mean, look at me with that Doctor Vashraf.'

I had to laugh. Vashraf was a kind and gentle Muslim who spent more time in observing Islamic rites than he did in helping Manners to whom he was supposed to be an assistant. When he wasn't praying or meditating he was in the kitchen preparing food for himself. In fact, the domestic staff had been so peeved they'd threatened to bring the union in, and Vashraf had been forbidden to enter the kitchen because, as the domestic supervisor told him, doctors were easy to get and cooks weren't.

'Ever since then Vashraf's been in a right old sulk. I think he's applied for other jobs because I've seen him several times walking down the avenue in his best suit. So whatever there may be about Stafford's murky past, if I were you, I'd make all the hay you can.'

That was what I intended to do, I said, and was about to get up and go down to St Basil's when Manners snapped his fingers.

'I knew I'd something else to ask you. Have you ever

come across a wild social worker called Pillsworth?'

I laughed and told him about the Dippy episode.

'Well, I was on call with her the other week. After calling me out and asking my opinion, she then goes against me. Now you know I get on well with Social Services, after all my wife's a social worker, but this woman's a menace.'

'What did she do?' I laughed, Manners looked so indignant.

'What did she do? After getting me out to see a Mrs Ainsworth, who's had a pattern of going into manias for years now . . .'

I knew Mrs Madge Ainsworth, I interrupted. She was my patient. And when she went mad it was in the good old-fashioned, florid way that you didn't see so much of today, what with the new drugs and treatments.

'Right. Well, Nurse Milligan . . .'

'The head of the Community Nurses team?'

'That's it. Maggie Milligan had seen Mrs Ainsworth a few days ago and thought she needed admission. The GP, Doctor Waters, was all for it because Madge kept phoning him to ask where the crown jewels were . . .'

'That's Madge. She usually thinks she's the Queen.'

'Right. Anyway, after spending an hour with the Queen I wanted to sign a section to commit her to Barrington and this Pillsworth woman says the time isn't ripe and that really, in spite of the delusions and hallucinations, Mrs Ainsworth wasn't harming anyone and she, Miss Pillsworth, would call every day and keep an eye on her. Doctor Waters was so mad he phoned Miss P, and do you know she gave him hell about human rights and needs. Waters reminded her that he'd been in practice when she was only a uterine blob and who the hell did she think she was? He's going to report her to the Director of Social Services.'

It was right and good that so much care was taken over enforced admission to mental hospitals. I saw nothing wrong with the system which made it necessary for social workers to have to make the application for the admission of patients as well as doctors. But many doctors resented this as usurping their powers and Kate Pillsworth, with her dogmatic attitude, didn't help. The establishing of a new profession like social work into a working relationship with an old and conservative profession like medicine, called for tact on both sides, and I knew that Monty Waters, with his rather pompous manner and stubborn, old-fashioned views, was the type to have a very low rage-threshold with clumsy young women like Kate.

'She's well meaning,' I said, 'but her manner is unfortunate and tactless. Madge Ainsworth won't last, her mania will escalate and she'll have to come into hospital.'

'I know that,' Manners growled. 'But that bloody woman Pillsworth, by her pig-headed attitude, has delayed treatment. She needs certifying herself.'

I met Oliver outside the canteen. He was chatting to Nurse Whelan, a blue-eyed blonde on Flower Ward. Her head thrown back, she was laughing at something Stafford was saying. When he spoke you felt he was directing laser-like attention to what you were saying, and he had the Welsh articulacy. So as well as academic ability there was this ease and grace of manner which could only be described by the hackneyed word 'charm'. I asked him whether he'd like to come to the clinic with me as I knew he'd finished with the ward work in the hospital. He'd probably have time on his hands till he collected some more patients at the clinic, I told him on the way down to St Basil's.

'I can always find something to do,' he said. 'And I'm doing a paper on phobias which involves quite a bit of reading. Meantime, I hope you don't mind my sitting in with you for today.'

Not at all, I said, two shrinks were better than one.

Doctor Gillespie had done his stuff with Wendy Cotton and had managed to get her to come to see me. While Sister bustled off to fetch her in, I ran over her background with

Oliver. She was a desperate and distraught girl, I explained, an insecure and unhappy childhood had made her very vulnerable to stress and her infertility, newly discovered, had shattered her.

Stafford stared at me with those tawny, intent eyes and said, 'I can imagine. Olwyn and myself have that problem. We'd have loved a family but it seems it's not going to happen . . .' He shrugged and looked away.

So, there might be marital troubles I thought, but he neutered this idea by adding that they had learned to live with it and maybe they'd adopt when they were more 'settled'. I hadn't time to dwell on this theory because Wendy came in.

'This is Doctor Stafford, Wendy. Do you mind him being here?'

She shook her head. The agitation was less because Doctor Gillespie had put her on some Valium. Her movements were slow and languid as she pushed some wispy brown hair out of her sad eyes. Whereas before she'd been as taut as a violin string, today she was retarded. Her voice was slow and thickened and she spoke in a monosyllabic way. She was as depressed as ever, it was as deep as last time, but now it showed itself in slow retardation. There were no more outbursts of despair; no thrashing of her thin limbs; no tears in the dull eyes, she just wasn't with us. Again, I asked her would she not come into hospital, but she shook her head in weary dissent.

'A sick child,' said Oliver, when she had left after agreeing to come and see me next week. 'If it weren't for the retardation I'd say she was suicidal.'

I was about to agree when the phone rang. Damn! I'd forgotten I was on duty. As if that wasn't enough it was Kate Pillsworth on the line. Predictably, Mrs Ainsworth was on the rampage.

Madge had barricaded herself in the house and was running up a huge telephone bill by continuously ringing her loyal subjects. The neighbours on both sides had complained to the police because of the phone calls from Madge and their very real concern that Mrs Ainsworth would beggar herself.

'Well, of course, if Madge had come into hospital before this we could have started her treatment. She always recovers in a few weeks after some electric treatment.'

'Isn't that a bit old-fashioned,' Kate said. 'I thought ECT had been given up?'

This was the sort of Pillsworth comment which maddened people. I said rather acidly that ECT was still used to advantage in selected cases, and Madge Ainsworth was one of them.

'I was wondering if you could come along to try to perduade Mrs Ainsworth to come into hospital?' Miss Pillsworth asked.

'But, Miss Pillsworth, if Madge is refusing to come out of her house, how do you propose we get her into hospital? By throwing a committal order through the letter box?'

Oliver lifted his eyebrows and I could feel my voice getting edgier and edgier.

'Well, I'm sorry I had to disagree with Doctor Manners but, you see, I wanted to give Mrs Ainsworth a chance to come in of her own volition. I didn't think she was a danger to herself or others at that time, but now I think she is . . .'

'Only none of us can get in to do anything about it. I still think it's a pity Madge wasn't sent in to hospital before things got to this stage. Right. I'll be along.'

I asked Stafford whether he wanted to get home and he said not at all, he'd come with me to see Madge.

Madge Ainsworth lived in a very salubrious part of Yorkely, all tree-lined private roads, and a favourite haunt of target thieves and burglars. The Berries was a noble looking house in red brick and hidden by the holly trees which gave it it's name.

Miss Pillsworth came striding to the car, her face flushed and her bronze hair standing out like a furze bush. 'Sorry to have to call,' she said, 'but I've been here for two hours and I can't do anything to get her out. She's standing in the hall telephoning all the time and, the GP says, running up huge bills.'

We walked towards the front of the ivy-covered old house and I banged on the heavy oak door. I didn't expect any response but to my surprise the door flew open and there was Madge. Usually, when she was well, she was a fastidious old lady who kept herself immaculately, spending time and money on her make-up, hair and clothes. Now, her white hair was screwed into ratty-looking plaits, her face hollow with fatigue and her grubby old dressing gown, tied together with a safety pin, had egg stains on it. Normally Madge would have collapsed with horror at using a pin to keep her gown together, but now she was in high mania, her brain racing wildly and her behaviour lacking any brake of wisdom or sensitivity. Due to the blunting of sensibility that a derangement like mania brings, she had lost all her former cultivation, and a coarser, blunted persona took over. The malevolent eyes and the drawn back, dry lips were a cruel mask of Madge's normal, gentle expression.

'No tradesmen, please,' she snarled, and banged the door in my face.

I peeped through the letter box and saw her go back to the phone by the heavy chest in the dark, tiled hall.

'Six bottles of brandy and some cigars,' she was saying. Then she went on to china tea and special mints.

How terrible, Miss Pillsworth whispered. Madge would have no money left. I forbore rubbing in the fact that if Madge had been sent in to Barrington before this we'd all have been saved much bother, and poor Madge wouldn't be running up debts. I said I'd have another go at trying to persuade her to let us in so, again I began to coax her through the letter box.

'Just a moment, one of my subjects wants an audience,' I heard her say, then the door was unlocked and Madge appeared again. Before I could say or do anything she shouted at me to 'piss off' in most unregal tones.

Kate looked put out. The people next door had told her that Mrs Ainsworth used most unqueenly language when she was ill. Last night, apparently, Madge had stalked out to the back garden and begun roaring some lewd ditties. The police had been called but hadn't wanted to get involved, especially when they heard that Madge had been in Barrington Hall.

'It's a matter of getting at Mrs Ainsworth so that we can make out the committal order,' Kate said uncertainly.

'We can't do it through the letter box,' I snapped, biting back a great temptation to say I told you so, and reminded Kate that all this present trouble could have been avoided.

'And the GP is getting fed up with Mrs Ainsworth phoning him out of hours,' Kate went on. 'There are no relatives of course, which makes it more difficult.'

That was true. Madge was the widow of a High Court judge and I wondered what Judge Clement Ainsworth would have to say about the present goings on.

My ruminations were interrupted by the sound of the door being thrown open. Madge appeared looking very angry and pointing a hand in our direction. Her stained gown parted to reveal a bosom down which toilet paper had been stuffed. 'Ignorant scum! If you all aren't off the palace grounds in two seconds I'll set my corgis on you.'

The corgis were no more than one obese pekinese who was hardly able to waddle due to overfeeding, let alone set about anyone. As the door slammed, Oliver said he'd have a go at persuading Madge.

Kate and I retreated. Had she heard any more of Mr Dippy? Not a word, she replied. She'd called back twice to the house and although she was met with pleased smiles from the Indian lodgers, she hadn't been able to find out what had become of Dippy. Probably beat it back to Pakistan, I said, after the traumatisation of the pork chop. Kate smiled rather slowly, humour wasn't very prominent in her make-up.

Stafford stepped back from the door. He'd been talking to Madge through the letter box. The door opened and Madge tripped out. Oliver spoke to her, then they linked arms and walked towards us.

'Her Majesty has consented to come with us for a rest,' Oliver said gravely, and Madge looked at us with haughty condescension.

'What about her clothes?' I asked. 'And Porky the dog?'

'I'll see to that,' Kate Pillsworth said. 'And we can do the papers at the hospital.'

'I'll sign no pardons for you two,' Madge shrilled. Lucky it was so warm this end of a May day. Her tatty gown was frayed and thin, and the dingy nightie underneath was torn. Her feet and hands were black with dirt.

'Well done,' I said to Oliver as he and Mrs Ainsworth got into the back of the car. Kate Pillsworth, who had the key to the house, would follow later to the hospital.

As Madge gabbled away in a rambling, discursive fashion, I felt very pleased that we had managed to get her to come to the hospital. We would sedate her first and then repair her dehydration and starvation. That, just repairing the fluid loss in old, neglected people, was often dramatically successful in restoring calm. A few days of being looked after worked miracles with Madge, and after four weeks or less she would be back home in The Berries with an amnesia for her psychosis and a restoration of the graciousness of the real Madge Ainsworth.

When we got back to the hospital we handed Madge over to the nurses and Oliver said he'd stay and examine her. I was going to remind him that she normally required pretty heavy sedation when I remembered that that would perhaps be insulting to someone with his clinical acumen.

He'd be grateful, he said, if I would just pop in and tell Olwyn that he'd be late.

'Not guilty,' I said later to Olwyn. Her husband wasn't even on duty. He'd insisted on staying to examine the patient. I didn't want her to think I was a slave driver, I said, and she laughed. She had a very loud laugh, almost raucous for someone so ethereal and she threw her head back.

'He'll never change, Oliver. And I tell him, I say, "Oliver you're not in your twenties any more you know. Slow down . . ."'

I wondered what age he was. In spite of Olwyn's friendliness I couldn't ask her anything as personal as that. From the entry in the medical register and his date of qualification I'd put him in his mid-thirties. And she?

'I'm six years older than him, you know. But I was a duffer at school and he was so bright that by the end of schooldays Oliver had floated to the top of the class. We were very proud of him in the village, you know. He got a scholarship to Cardiff University.'

'Yes. I could see by his record that he was honours material,' I said.

'You looked him up then? Naturally. Yes, he did very well, Oliver. Of course he's not ambitious, not trying to prove anything or break any records. He always wanted to be a doctor and he loves everything about the job. He's not ruthless enough to be a good competitor, having to walk over bodies and kick away rungs; all the rotten things you have to do to get on, well they're just not in my husband's nature. The price of seniority is too high, that's what Oliver says.'

She sounded quietly triumphant and I was sure she was telling me this to answer the questions she must have known I'd be asking. And maybe I was too quick to look for complications and elaborations when simplicity was the clue. Olwyn's next words seemed to confirm this.

'We're just two country bumpkins at heart, Oliver and me. I guess we'll end up in a Welsh village with Oliver delivering babies and me lambs. I must go, Joyce, I hear something boiling over.'

Next day, when I got to St Basil's, I saw Wendy Cotton, hunched and miserable looking, like Little Orphan Annie in her too-big dress. Lee Kelly, the young psychologist who had treated Wendy successfully for her stammer, had phoned me earlier in the day to ask about her. Lee had heard that Wendy was ill again and was wondering if there was anything she could do. I liked Lee, she was as nice as she was clever and she'd certainly been patient and caring with Wendy, using conditioning and behaviour therapy to rid the girl of her speech impediment so well that I forgot Wendy had ever stammered. Now the trouble was for the girl to try to accept her sterility.

'Sterile? But Wendy loves kids. She kept telling me how keen she was to have a child of her own.'

'That's out,' I said. 'And she's taking it badly.'

'I can understand that,' said Lee, who told me she was pregnant herself.

That news wouldn't help poor Wendy who looked abject when she came in, lost and enclosed in a private hell.

'Tell me, Wendy,' I asked, 'how is your husband taking this? Will he be able to come here with you next week?'

'What for?'

'Well, I'd like to discuss things with him. See what he feels. About not having kids and about you.'

'I dunno. It's hard for him to get off work. I told you, he's all right, Ron. He says he's not worried.'

'But surely he's worried about you?'

I always liked to see the two partners of a marriage if I was treating one. For one thing it was useful to know if the spouse, who wasn't obviously ill, cared enough about their partner to come to the clinic with them and, for another, it didn't make sense to treat a husband or wife as a unit rather than a partner.

'He's a good bloke,' Wendy said. 'Too good to be tied to someone like me. I dunno why you bother with me,' she went on. 'What can you do? There's plenty of people outside sicker than me. Everyone's got problems haven't they? That's life, I reckon. Last week when I was waiting I saw a man brought in on a stretcher and his legs was all crushed after an accident and he screamed and cried something awful. He kept groaning, "It hurts, it hurts," and you could see the blood coming through the bandages. Now he was really ill. Not like me.'

'But you are ill, Wendy. It's just that the blood isn't showing and when someone says to you, "Show me where it hurts," you can't point to any one spot. So don't think you're wasting my time. I don't think I am, otherwise I wouldn't see you. Try and bring your husband along with you next week.'

She went out, slouching, her back bowed like an old woman and a Mrs Estelle Hawks was shown in. Her address was in the road Mrs Ainsworth lived in and from what I knew of the referring GP, Doctor Gordon Grimes, he had mostly private patients, but the reasons for his referring Mrs Hawks to me soon became obvious.

She sat down, crossed her legs and stared at me coolly. She was a very attractive woman, her skin lightly tanned against the cream of her very expensively cut trouser suit. Aquamarine eyes and dark blonde hair streaked in places. Her slim hands clanked with gold bracelets as she flicked at a gold cigarette lighter.

'Doctor Grimes says in his letter, Mrs Hawks, that you want a termination. How many months are you pregnant?'

'Over two. It's all a bit vague. Didn't think I was pregnant at first, especially as my youngest child is fifteen.'

It couldn't be that she was physically ill. She looked glowingly healthy with the sort of gleam and patina that only money and time can achieve.

'So there is a psychiatric reason for termination?'

The turquoise eyes were now more green than blue and her face changed to a sulky resentment.

'Look. I didn't come here to be interrogated. Are you a Catholic?'

'Yes. But that's irrelevant. You see, you just can't walk in, to me anyway, and say you want an abortion. There has to be danger to the mother or child.'

'I didn't want to come here in the first place, waiting outside with all those loonies. I knew Grimes wanted to fob me off. And to tell me that you can't get an abortion just like that is rubbish, Doctor.'

She nearly spat the last word at me and I could see that she wasn't as young as I had thought. Frowning and cross, the make-up stood out more, especially around the eyes.

'I can walk into the Harvey Clinic here in Yorkely and get an abortion just like that,' she continued, snapping her fingers derisively at me. 'I only came here because it's holiday period and Grimes couldn't get me seen elsewhere in a hurry. I tell you, I can't have this baby. It's not on. And I *won't* have it.'

Then she should have been more careful with her contraception I nearly said. After poor Wendy's sorrow I was beginning to seethe at this rich bitch and I had a job keeping a very raw edge out of my voice.

'My husband can afford to pay for me privately,' Mrs Hawks said, stubbing out her cigarette as if she were grinding it to pieces. 'Just my luck to get a nosey woman,' she added, green eyes flashing.

'Tell me, Mrs Hawks,' I said. 'Just why do you want an abortion? You are healthy, sane, assure me that you have money. Why *don't* you want the baby?'

She stood up, tossed the blonde hair back and swung her

soft leather shoulder-bag over one silk-clad shoulder.
'Because we're going to the South of France next month and
I want to wear my bikini.'

'If that's your reason then I agree you aren't fit to be a
mother at all!' The words just flew out of my mouth in spite
of such small restraint as was natural to me.

She banged the door so hard that Sister raced in to see
what was the matter!

Chapter Seven

June was like May. Indeed the weather was even more clement and everyone who could get away did so, making the work with the patients even more difficult because their flow never stopped and if anything they increased in numbers. But having Oliver made a tremendous difference to me. His earlier industry wasn't just a fluke, or the planned policy of the alcoholic or drug addict to create a good impression that would stand him in good stead when he broke out later. He was naturally keen on medicine and psychiatry and his ability to get on with people made him very popular with staff as well as patients. Even Frankie was coming around to the opinion that Felix, whatever his motivation, had done me and the hospital a bit of good.

Although Coulter hadn't bothered to say a formal farewell he had given an embarrassingly cloying speech at the farewell sherry party in his office where, after accepting a gold clock from us, his medical colleagues, he waxed almost poetical about how sorry he was to leave us and how much he'd miss us. Manners and myself deduced this sloppy sentimentality was brought on by too much sweet sherry and the presence of Mrs Coulter, huge in trailing chiffon, and a bandeau on her hair.

'I shall have to pop off soon, got bit more packing to do. So I'll say cheerio.' Coulter loomed up behind Manners and myself.

'I hope the advertisement for your replacement has gone in,' Manners said sharply.

'Should have. Stafford still working hard, Joyce?'

'His energy reminds me of the far off days when I first qualified,' I said. 'He actually seems to enjoy his work.'

Coulter beamed. To enjoy work was becoming a rarity in the battered NHS. He was delighted that I found Stafford a help, he knew Oliver would fit in as soon as he saw him and, of course, he'd had a very good recommendation from Haxton Hospital.

'Why did he leave Haxton, then?'

It was such an obvious question that I was surprised to see how Coulter became so evasive. He stared over to where Oliver was standing chatting to Mrs Coulter who looked massively handsome in navy and white. She was showing a lot of teeth, waving her cigarette holder and flirting with Oliver. 'Oh, I gather Stafford's a bit of a rolling stone. Itchy feet,' Felix replied.

I was diverted from following up this rather cryptic remark by seeing Olwyn come in on her own. She looked dreamy in a white dress made of a drifting material. Her beauty had nothing of the bouncing outdoor girl type; she would look best away from the sun, rather like a victorian maiden with the sort of huge-eyed pallidity which often indicated consumption.

'Over here, Olwyn,' I called.

I could see Oliver hadn't spotted her, and she smiled gratefully at me. The way she was wearing her hair today, two wings framing her face, for some reason reminded me of a gentle dove.

'Have you met Mrs Stafford?' I asked. 'Doctor Felix Coulter.'

She murmured something and Felix jiggled uncomfortably. He was always bad socially and today he seemed more boorish than ever. He'd have to get back to his wife who seemed to be beckoning to him. From my vantage point, I couldn't see any such thing. Mrs Coulter was accepting another sherry and laughing at something Oliver was saying. He in turn, had seen Olwyn and was waving to her.

'We've so much to do . . . crates . . . packing . . . finalising the house sale . . .' Coulter really was not his normal apparently placid self.

'I can't understand Doctor Coulter,' I said. 'It must be the thought of America that's making him so edgy. Look at the way he's rushing his wife out. You'd think he'd wait for the end of his own party.'

Olwyn went over to join her husband and I began to talk to Cissie Bates, a visiting anaesthetist who did some sessions at Barrington. I rather liked Cissie, she was tall and very dark and dashing in an avant garde fashion. Today she was wearing a very elegant lily-green shift and carried an alligator bag that matched her shoes. She was dying to be bitchy about the Coulters because she didn't like Felix, whose lack of style and boringly tedious conversation offended her own good taste.

'I saw Felix doing an ill-mannered bolt,' she said. 'He'll go down well in the States he's so brash. I was standing behind Mrs Coulter and she was having a delightful time vamping Doctor Stafford, dropping her handbag and her aitches. They're an attractive couple.'

'The Coulters?'

'Don't be ridiculous. No, I mean the Staffords. I hear he's a tremendous worker. Strange he hasn't done more, had a better job by now.'

'That's what I can't understand,' I said. 'With his ability and experience I'd have thought he'd have gone places. Of course, he was spotted by Coulter at Haxton Hospital and that's another mystery; why didn't he stay? He wasn't getting more seniority by coming to us, and Felix was evasive when I asked him.'

'Oh, Coulter loves the cloak and dagger stuff. Likes to be the Great Fixer. I shouldn't worry too much, Joyce. You needed help and assistance and now you've got it, so relax and enjoy it.'

'Just what I always say.' Doctor Tony Manners appeared. He was quite a favourite of Cissie because he could turn on the gallantry that she enjoyed. In spite of being in her forties and a dedicated career woman, Cissie adored men and had been the subject of much gossip when younger.

I looked over to where the Staffords were talking together. They certainly seemed happy and relaxed, with none of the unease in each other's company indicative of marital strain. I should go over and join them but there was something on my mind. Coulter's job would be free now. Why shouldn't Oliver have a crack at it? After all, we knew him to some extent, and certainly his work couldn't be faulted. He hadn't shown any alarming vices and was strictly a one drink man, he'd told me. I should sound him out, discover whether he felt like staying in Yorkely. Better still, I could sound Olwyn out.

I got an opportunity to this some days later. I was coming home at about six o'clock and I could see Olwyn doing something at the sink in her kitchen which looked out over the garden. Charlie, the crusty old patient who worked so hard in the garden was leaning on his spade. He'd always been ill and irascible with me. So much so that I left him alone, putting up with his paranoid mutterings and ferocious glares because he was a marathon worker and had made the old garden into such a well cared for and colourful place. But ever since the Staffords arrived he had become a different man. He was actually grinning now as he limped over to me with a basket of flowers for Olwyn. The limp was another reason I put up with him; he'd been a Dunkirk victim and had sustained several bullets in his leg which left him maimed.

'I don't know what spell you've put on Charlie,' I said to Olwyn, handing her the basket.

'He's a dear. An old pet. We have long chats. Won't you come in for a few moments. I'd just made tea for Charlie and there's enough in the pot if you want a cup?'

I thanked her and declined. But I'd like a few words with her, I said, following her indoors.

'Sure. You don't mind me carrying on with supper preparations?'

'Not at all,' I replied.

She went back to the sink and her hands began to fly, tossing lettuce, slicing cucumber and chopping carrots. 'Isn't this summer wonderful? It's the sort of weather we think happened all the time in childhood. Sure you wouldn't like some wine? Oliver has some rather good grapefruit wine that he made last year? Or there's some sherry?'

No sherry, I said, but I'd like to ask her something.

She tossed back her dark brown hair, long and loose today, and began to whisk some salad dressing in a bowl. 'Ask away.'

Maybe I should have spoken to Oliver first, I said, and maybe I was talking out of turn, but did they like Yorkely? Did Oliver like working in Barrington?

'Oh, yes. Very much. And I like my job. Everything's going too well for us. Really well.'

Did I detect relief in her tone? It seemed to me that the way she emphasised the 'really well' was important. Had something happened in Haxton? I'd have to stop being so suspicious, Coulter was right about my being too probing. As Cissie said, the thing to do was to relax and enjoy it.

'What it is,' I went on, plunging right in, 'now you're settled here, in the flat and everything, I was wondering whether Oliver was interested in staying for a bit? There are two jobs coming up, one is a consultant's, Coulter's job in fact. I don't know whether Oliver could get that but I'm pretty sure he'd have a chance of the registrar's job. That's if he's interested.'

She whirled around, clapping her hands so hard the cat leaped down from one of the chairs where he'd been lying like a black fur stole. 'Oh, yes. The answer is yes. If Oliver has a chance I'm sure he'd love to stay. He likes the job, likes working with you.'

Now then, here goes, I thought and I said, 'I have to ask

you something, Olwyn. And I don't want to ask Oliver. But, obviously, if Oliver wants to go for a job here we'd have to ask for a reference from Haxton.'

The words were out, dropped just like that and I knew Olwyn was upset by the way she came over to the table and sat down. She said nothing for a while and I thought Christ, I've stirred something. There's going to be stalling, revelations or a polite request for me to mind my own business.

'Of course, of course. It's the obvious question, isn't it? The one people ask with their eyes but are too polite to voice. So I'll tell you . . .'

'Not if it hurts you to. I really only asked you because we couldn't not have a reference. And the obvious place to ask is Oliver's last hospital.'

Silence again and Olwyn stared down at her clasped hands. How small they were, like a child's, pale and almost pudgy with very short nails.

'I'd like to tell you the whole story. I will some day. Anyway, you'll find that they thought Oliver was tops at Haxton. The reason we left is because of me. Something I did. Not Oliver. You mustn't think it's his fault . . .'

I was rigid with embarrassment, furious that I'd got involved in soul baring and frightened of what she was going to tell me.

'You must believe me. Oliver would have stayed at Haxton, if it wasn't for me. I'm not a girl for cosy confidences,' she said.

I wasn't one for spiritual strip-tease myself, I replied. But I still wondered why she was so preoccupied in sheltering Oliver.

'Let's just say then that it was my fault we left Haxton. Nothing to do with Oliver and his job. And of course there are lots of places which will give him references. Left to himself he'd have stayed there. Oh, yes, I know he's been a wanderer up until now, we both liked to be on the move.

Comes a time though when you want to stay put, put down a few roots, and this is the stage we've reached. We want to stay and work here and make a go of things . . .' I sensed she was trying to tell me something.

The kitchen was made rosy by the setting sun and Olwyn sat, lost in her own thoughts, so quiet that both of us jumped when Oliver tapped at the window. I was glad to see him, glad that the strain of Olwyn's outburst was dissipated by Oliver who was amused by what a patient's daughter had told him about her mother.

'That she was "intercontinental", so much nicer than "incontinent". Have you asked Joyce to taste the wine, Olwyn? D'you know we began to make liqueurs but got so fond of them we were turning into two old tipplers.'

I thanked him but refused the wine. Whether he noticed Olwyn's strained appearance and my embarrassment I don't know, but he seemed full of bounce and cheerfulness and I left him taking a turn at whisking the salad dressing.

Frankie called on me later. She'd been making a call quite near to the Priest's House and was on her way home. I told her what Olwyn had said and she thought about it, chewed it up and turned it round with her usual appreciation of people's foibles.

'Well, there you have it. The Welsh are a sexy lot, you know. Wonder who the man was?' she asked.

'What man?'

'Olwyn's lover. You can't very well have an affair without one.'

'She didn't say that. She didn't come right out and tell me that she was having an affair and that's why they left Haxton.'

'She said it was her fault, didn't she?'

'Just that. No more. She told me that it certainly wasn't anything to do with Oliver.'

'Then what the hell else could it be but that our Olwyn

had herself an affair. God knows, Oliver must spend enough time away from her, maybe neglects her while he does some strenuous hunting on his own. So she has herself a little fling. Maybe with one of the Haxton staff, some nice young houseman or maybe that Doctor Johnson, the big guy with the streaked hair. I've heard a thing or two about him. Apparently his wife's lesbian and . . .'

She was off, frolicking over the fascinating possibilities, till I got a fit of yawning and Frankie said she had to go. She'd forgotten that she'd bought cigars for Barney who'd be fuming as he waited for them. At the door she paused and said she'd ask the Staffords over for a meal this Saturday. And I was to come, too. Fine by me, I said, and she dashed off. Then she raced back up the stairs and said that Barney wasn't too well and could we make it Saturday week? That seemed all right, I said, and asked what was wrong with Barney.

'He's got a gastric upset, it's lasting a long time. Makes him mumpish and he shouldn't be smoking, but what can I do? I'll be in touch with you soon.'

The following week started with a bang when I was phoned by the local police to say that they were holding a woman who'd been a patient of mine, Mrs Vivaleen Cider.

'We've had the Police Surgeon who thinks Mrs Cider is needing Barrington. D'you recall her, Doctor?'

Could I ever forget Vivaleen? A large, rollicking West Indian woman in her forties, she was a fervent Pentecostal and was so immersed in her own peculiar religiosity that she forgot to take her tablets and so at times, rather like Mrs Ainsworth, went into roaring mania which took the form of delusions that she was seeing and hearing God, on a hot line to Him in fact. Added to which she threw in some weird bits of voodoo, the St Kitt's variety.

I could hear the well-known bellow of Vivaleen belting out a hymn, and PC Wiggin sounded hushed as he said the sedative the police doctor had ordered didn't seem to be working, and please would I come as soon as I could?

I could vouch for that. Vivaleen, due to her size and the roistering strength of her mania, needed blockbuster doses of tablets. Mega-Therapy as Tony Manners had it.

I was always in a bit of a flurry trying to park my car in front of Framley police station after there had been an embarassing episode last year when I'd scraped a visiting CID man's car. I could hear Mrs Cider almost as soon as I stepped on to the station. Three young policemen had a job to contain their chortles, and as one of them showed me to the cell where Vivaleen had been placed he beamed and said he wouldn't like my job if I had to deal with people like Mrs Cider. The young policewoman sitting with Vivaleen looked pale and rumpled. Her hair was coming loose from its neat bun and her white shirt was parting from the band of her black skirt.

'Doctor D. Am I glad to see you.'

Vivaleen threw her arms around me and smacked kisses on my face. She smelt of sweat, onions and barley wine. She wore a short red dress encasing her like the skin of a sausage, her bare, black legs were stuck into Minnie Mouse white court shoes which had bulged under her weight and her mass of fuzzy Afro-style hair stood out from her enormous smiling face.

'I hear ya Lard. Keep it comin'. Amen. Hallelujah!' She cupped a huge black hand behind one ear and adopted a listening attitude. The young policewoman skipped away from Vivaleen's suddn lunge and the big woman threw back her head and laughed roaringly. 'No need to be scared of Vivaleen, police lady. I jus' want peace and love. Peace and love.'

The policeman who had shown me to the bleak cell stayed beside his colleague and they both looked embarrassed and scared, something which Vivaleen, who had an animal sense of who was scared of her, saw quite clearly. She began to stamp up and down in the cell bellowing a bawdy calypso.

'Isn't she a terror?' the policewoman whispered. She was staring at the large woman as if she was a Martian.

'Thousan's have been and there's room for thousan's more,' roared Vivaleen, swinging her white bag as if it was a drum stick.

'What's all this then?' The large, whiskery policeman who had appeared was evidently senior and said sharply that Vivaleen could be heard all over the station and the detectives trying to interview a suspect had complained of the din.

Fortunately, Bob Morris from Social Services arrived and he was quiet and efficient and, best of all, knew Vivaleen and could handle her. 'Best to get her straight up to the hospital,' he whispered.

I said to Vivaleen that she needed a rest and attention, and we wanted her to come into hospital.

'No way, Doc darlin'. No way.' She began to strut again and resumed her lewd song, while the senior of the policemen adjusted his helmet and looked cross.

'Now, stop showing off, Vivaleen,' I said. 'The Lord wants you to come with us. He's told me so.'

'What the Lard want then Vivaleen do.' Mrs Cider stopped her pacing and gave a huge flash of her white teeth.

'She's like a female version of Mohammed Ali,' the young policeman murmured. 'Fly like a butterfly and sting like a bee.'

But Vivaleen was anything but a butterfly and when the policewoman, still looking scared, opened the cell and Mrs Cider trundled out she grabbed at the policewoman and lifted her up in the air.

'Now then,' the helmeted policeman shot forward and roughly tried to prise the terrified girl away from the arms of

Vivaleen. With a raucous laugh Vivaleen knocked off his helmet, and two more policemen appeared as the furious copper retrieved his helmet.

'That shook ya, whitey!' Vivaleen burst into loud laughter, but when Bob Morris linked her arm she took it quietly enough and went off with him.

'D'you get many like that?' the shaken looking police-woman asked, as she rearranged her crooked black tie and stared down at her torn and laddered black tights. 'I'd rather face an Aston Villa match than that woman!'

Part of the job, I said, as we walked up the stone passage and back to the front of the station. There was a smell of dust and ink and a lingering suggestion of Dettol, used I supposed to clean up after people like Vivaleen. A policeman in black trousers and a blue shirt was taking particulars from a small man in a shabby mac who was leaning over the counter waving a burned out cigarette to emphasise what he was saying. The policeman seated at the telephone was asking whoever was on the other end to please speak up. I caught the name he was asking to be spelled.

'M for man, E for end, L for letter, I for item, N for not, D for dog, A for apple . . . Boden.' The policeman was wiring carefully on a pad. 'I've got the particulars. We'll contact you just as soon as we hear anything . . .'

I stopped, frozen, and asked what that was about, that message. Because I knew a Sheena Boden, in fact, she was a patient of mine.

'Well. I'm afraid she's in trouble, Doc. Her child is missing. She went into Marks and Spencer's in Yorkely, left the child in a passage and when she came out the kid was gone . . .'

There had to be an explanation, I said, Melinda could have walked away, she could toddle quite well.

'No. The mother said she strapped her in securely because of that. The kid's stroller was left. I gather the mother hasn't been well, Doctor?'

That was putting it mildly, I said. Knowing Sheena I could vouch that she'd made the child secure. I must get round there right away, I gabbled.

'Hate these cases,' PC Wiggin said. 'I've got three kids of me own. This had to be some paranoid nut or . . .'

He didn't have to finish, we both knew the amount of paedophiles there were in Yorkely.

'You will try and help, won't you? This child is so precious. The mother's whole world.'

'Every child's precious,' Wiggin reproved me gently. 'I can promise you we'll do our best. Can I have your telephone number, too?'

After I'd given it to him I drove quickly to Sheena's. The shock had driven away much of the improvement of the past few weeks. She stood, hands hanging by her side and her face agonised.

'I tried to get you. I should have brought her in with me. Shouldn't have left her. I feel . . . feel as if I've had . . . I feel as if my heart's been torn out. I keep thinking. Not so much about who took her as how she is.'

There was nothing to say, nothing of any real comfort to this poor distraught girl who had so very little in life, and now her small link with sanity and happiness had been taken. I put my arm around Sheena and told her the string of useless clichés I was telling myself. I'd been in the police station when she'd been on the line. The police were very good at finding missing persons, especially when it was a child. Many of them were fathers themselves. So she mustn't, mustn't give up hope.

'There's something else; I keep thinking of it. It's like a worm eating at my brain. You know, you read about these sick people . . . perverts I think they're called, who rape children. I'm always seeing things like that in the paper. What if . . .?' She stared at me, her eyes glazed and fixed, her jaw dropping in sick horror. 'Why? Why? Haven't I suffered enough?'

I could see resemblances to the crazed girl who'd had her reality shattered by schizophrenia, now she was having to cope with a reality that was just as frightening as she'd had when she was ill. She wasn't crying, couldn't probably, her grief was too deep but her slack face and staring eyes were like those of someone who'd been involved in a major accident.

After I'd managed to persuade Sheena to have some of the tea I'd made, I asked her to come and stay the night with me. She didn't need much persuading and meekly swallowed the tranquillizer I gave her. To my surprise, and probably partly because she hadn't had to take sedation for ages now, Sheena was pole-axed by the drug and fell asleep with the light on.

'It'll probably hit her in the morning,' Frankie said when I phoned her. She was as sick and stunned at what had happened as I was. 'It'll send her diabetes all to hell and I hope it doesn't bring back her psychosis. What a bastard whoever took the child is. I hope to Christ the kid isn't found raped and strangled on some waste land.'

I could hear Barney shouting in the background and asked what he was saying.

'How sorry he is . . . he heard everything. So much for his deafness. Let me know immediately you hear anything. Oh . . . Barney wants a word.'

There was a crackling and loud cries of 'What the hell', and Barney came on the line. 'When they find the bugger that took the child . . . if they do . . . he'll probably trot out the usual excuse "something came over me". It never does when a policeman is near.'

Chapter Eight

Of course I didn't sleep. The night was hot and still and clammy, and even two baths didn't make me feel any cooler. Surprisingly, Sheena seemed to be in a very deep sleep every time I looked in at her. She lay, her arms flung out, with all the abandon of a child. When at last, towards dawn, I did manage to doze off I woke two hours later and I knew Sheena was awake because I could hear her sobbing. When I got up I found her huddled in a chair weeping.

'Oh, Sheena. Don't despair. I'm sure there'll be news today.'

She looked at me, her face raddled and ravaged, her eyes tortured pits. She said dully that that was what she was thinking about. There would probably be news that Mel was found dead.

'Listen. You think the worst. We all do. Let's keep hoping, love. I'll make some tea.'

She did manage to drink the tea but I couldn't get her to eat. I knew what she wanted me to do and I knew it was pointless to do it. The police would have rung if there was any news. It seemed too cruel to tell her, so I made the call to Framley and was lucky enough to get Policewoman Gilmore who said she was awfully sorry but there was no news, nothing at all. But everyone at the station was going all out to get a lead.

'How is the mother, poor kid?' Gilmore sounded like any concerned woman and she added that she was going on maternity leave herself at the end of the month. Yes, of course, they'd contact us when there was anything at all to report.

'Nothing?' Sheena asked dully, and I said no, not yet. She

dragged herself up with the heavy weariness of a tired, middle-aged woman and said she was going to have a bath.

Just then the door bell rang; it was Oliver. In spite of the sad circumstances and his obvious concern, I couldn't help noticing, maybe because of Sheena's torpidness, how relaxed and well he was looking.

'We've just heard about the Boden child. And Olwyn and I want to help in any way we can. Don't worry about the hospital. I'll see to it so you can stay here,' he said.

'But there's a new admission. Mrs Cider. I'll . . .'

He held up his hand. I wasn't to stir, he would see to things. O.K., I said, it was very good of him and I'd take him up on his offer because Sheena was staying with me and we didn't know when the phone would go wth news. I didn't have to explain anything, he said. 'Need any drugs? For sedation?'

No, I told him, I thought I had enough Valium, for the moment anyway. I didn't add what I was thinking, that Valium wouldn't be enough if the dreaded news came of a child's dead body being found. I was very conscious of Sheena hovering behind me. She was staring blankly at Oliver, her arms down by her sides, as if standing to attention. God alone knew what was going on in her drug-clouded brain. Oliver looked at her with a pity and compassion he seemed unable to express. He attempted to say something to her but then sighed hopelessly as she walked off to the bathroom.

'She looks like death,' he said, and I said yes, that was what I feared; this lack of news and the awful speculation it aroused was too much for her brittle nervous system. Oliver wished he could do more and I told him that his help with the work would be a Godsend.

The day was interminable. I was able to get Sheena to take Valium at least and although it made her drowsy the semi-sleep was restless and fretful. She drank fluids with persuasion but I couldn't get her to eat at all, and when she did nibble at some dry biscuits to please me, she vomited them back directly. She made me ring Framley station three times and when my phone rang at half past six in the evening she jumped in anguish. But it was only Olwyn apologising for not coming up to see us.

'One of the partners had to go to court unexpectedly and it's been so busy at the office. I'm so sorry I couldn't contact you sooner, Joyce. Any news?'

'No.'

'Now then, I've heated some soup and I can bring it up with some rolls.'

She was very kind but Sheena said she'd vomit again if she ate at the moment and as for me, well I had enough food in. Olwyn said please to phone her immediately if there was anything she could do and Oliver would cope tomorrow. He had arranged with Tony Manners to do my domiciliary calls. Before I could thank her and remind her to thank Oliver, she said she'd better get off the line in case anyone was trying to reach me. I had hardly put down the receiver when the phone rang again and poor Sheena sprang up, staring with a crazed sort of hope. But it was Frankie.

'I'm not going to ask how either of you are. I can imagine,' she said. 'Do you want me to come over? Bring food? Or stay the night?'

No. There was really nothing to be done other than grit the teeth, I said, which was easier for me than for poor Sheena.

'Quite. And the longer there's no news the more grim it becomes,' Frankie said. 'I cannot, just *cannot*, imagine the mentality of someone who'd do a thing like this. It's like people who plant bombs, they function at a sub-human level.'

I told her how supportive the Staffords were being. If Oliver wasn't here I would have had to go into the hospital, I couldn't farm out all my work.

'Yes, I think we have to take back our wild imaginings

about those two. Or at least if she has had an affair it doesn't mean she's not a nice person. That sounds Irish but you know what I mean. Barney sends his love.'

Another night, made a bit more bearable because I slept, and Sheena was still asleep when I got up and made the breakfast at eight o'clock. There was a rap at the door and old Charlie was there with my mail. That's funny. He'd never bothered before and then I realised that Oliver had probably sent him. Charlie looked as sour as ever but he told me he'd bring my letters again in the morning.

When I went to peep at Sheena at ten o'clock she woke quickly and sat up. I answered her silent question and said there had been no news.

'She must be dead,' Sheena moaned. 'What else could have happened? It's not kidnapping. The person who took her hasn't asked for money. I'm wondering whether I've done anything to anybody who's paying me back this way?'

It was as if all her tear ducts had dried up with inner agony. She shook with silent sobs and then dragged her hands through her matted, tangled hair. Now that she was undernourished and the strain was worsening, she had the taut, vulpine look that I remembered when she was so psychotically ill.

This present stressful agony could well precipitate another breakdown, I told Frankie when she rang before going to work. Sheena was in the bathroom so I explained to Frankie how low she was and how I feared a major crack-up again.

'God knows what this not eating is doing to her diabetes. Poor kid. She just doesn't deserve this does she? No wonder she's saying she must have done something to someone. Listen, I'll call in on the way home from work.'

At least the weather changed. Rain brought coolness and a welcome freshening of the air. My heart dead, I phoned the police. No, they hadn't heard anything and yes, things looked blacker. They had all the men and women they could spare working on the case but they'd come up with nothing. At the moment all the known peeping toms, flashers and child molesters were being vetted.

'In your experience, Constable Wiggin,' I asked, 'does the lack of clues indicate . . .' I just couldn't go further.

But Wiggin wasn't inhibited and he finished the sentence for me, 'The worst? Not really. We're bound to come up with something soon. How's the mother?'

'Bad,' I said, 'very bad.'

'Poor kid. Poor kid.'

We often said that the police weren't what they used to be. The young coppers hadn't the same feeling for the real relationship between the force and the local hospital. Two of the junior doctors had been done recently for speeding and they both said that when they told the police they were doctors it seemed to make things worse! But I was finding the Framley bunch to be in local Yorkshire parlance –'golden'.

The day creaked on and Sheena went back to bed. She lay curled in a ball, too tired for tears and even when the phone rang she didn't bother to get up. The strain would be bad enough for any mother, I told Frankie when she phoned later that afternoon, but in Sheena's case there was no supportive husband and a very tenuous and fragile grasp on sanity. The Valium, which I'd increased, was just holding her together.

I didn't hear Olwyn when she rang the door bell at six o'clock because I'd fallen into a fitful doze, and I came to with a sickening jerk, my body clammy with the sweat of fear.

Olwyn looked cool and fresh in an eau-de-nil dress and her long hair was tucked behind her ears. She carried a covered dish. 'I gathered neither of you would feel like eating something heavy, so as Charlie left us some salad things and raspberries I made a salad and a sort of mousse with the fruit.'

She was kind, I said. I wasn't hungry but her gesture touched me so much I made an effort to eat and was surprised to find that I was actually hungry. I was even more surprised when Sheena ate some of the raspberry mousse.

'Her first food in days,' I said. 'Let's try her with some coffee.'

'I'll make it,' said Olwyn and went into the kitchen.

Sheena let me wash her down with damp towels and then lay back on her pillows. Her long hair was scraggy and her face had fallen in, making her look twenty years older. She lay still and silent, not now bothering even too ask about news. I knew that she was resigned to the worst, that her child was dead, and she had withdrawn herself from the unbearable reality. The danger now was that she was on the point of toppling into her former black pit of psychotic despair, I told Olwyn, who sat down by the side of the bed and began to stroke the girl's waxy forehead. Slowly, slowly, she stroked and Sheena, although not appearing to be soothed and staring with glassy intensity, quite suddenly fell asleep.

'Let's have some coffee ourselves,' I whispered as we left the room.

When I handed Olwyn a cup of steaming liquid she said, 'You look half dead. Oliver says you're not to bother coming to the hospital tomorrow. He'll cope.'

'But I must. I can't cancel another clinic at St Basil's. No really, it's very good of Oliver but no, I'll come in. Only, if you could stay with Sheena? Is that all right?'

'No problem,' Olwyn replied. 'It's the very least I can do for you and for that poor girl next door. She seems half dead. I understand she was a patient of yours, Joyce? I hope this strain won't make her ill again?'

'There's every danger,' I said. 'Only this time she won't want to get better, if there's no Melinda to fight for.'

'It makes me ashamed. I have so much and she so little.'

Was she a bit too prone to denigrate herself? This was the

second time she'd seemed to be expressing guilt. Last time it was, as she said, 'all her fault' that Oliver hadn't settled down, and now here she was beating her breast again Funny girl. They said the Welsh were devious, maybe it was their sort of Celtic culture pattern? Then I was ashamed of my rather petty speculation. They'd both been so kind and helpful to me, I said, offering Olwyn more coffee.

'No thanks.' She shook her head. 'I'd better go down and get something for Oliver's supper. I'll be up here tomorrow at half past eight. Sure there's nothing more you need?' She paused interrogatively. She was like some dark beauty used to demonstrate some superior soap I thought. Serious, she was a little too remote looking, a sadness in the dark eyes, Mona Lisa before she middle-aged, but her smile lifted and lightened the pale face into a radiant luminosity. 'There's something I wanted to ask you, Joyce. Do you know anything about a Coralie Kane?'

'Why do you ask, Olwyn?'

'Well. She's phoned the house several times looking for Oliver. I just wondered what sort of woman she was?'

Something made me a bit guarded. Mrs Kane was a very neurotic and demanding patient, I said. I didn't add that I'd warned Oliver about Coralie. Surely he was able to handle her particular brand of manipulative behaviour? I didn't say this but I asked Olwyn whether Mrs Kane was being too much of a bother.

I didn't like the sound of this one little bit, Coralie phoning the Staffords' house. Of course it could just be part of the transaction between patient and therapist in which the client develops a positive transference for the doctor until the stage is resolved and cure comes about. I just didn't see this happening with Mrs Kane though, and neither did Olwyn, because she began to question me closely about Coralie, about her age, her appearance and so on until in the end I began to stall and tried to change the subject. Later, as if repenting her curiosity, Olwyn laughed and said she was ashamed to admit that she could be jealous of her husband.

On the way into my office at the clinic next afternoon, I could hear Coralie expounding to some fellow patients that it was all wrong the way they had to wait for me, I should have been here twenty minutes ago and she had a good mind to report me to the Ombudsman. Not that she minded, she had the good fortune to be under Doctor Stafford, who made up for his occasional lateness by giving her extra time at the end of the clinic. He was a real doctor, a born healer, you had only to look at his eyes; she wondered if he did hypnosis? Of course women doctors were a queer lot anyway. In fact, she was thinking of changing her GP who was a woman. She'd expected, Coralie said, to get an extra dimension of understanding from female doctors but she'd found they were impatient and waspish; they must be twisted up inside from doing a man's job. When she saw me she patted her confection of newly bleached hair and smiled falsely.

I would have to have words with Oliver about Coralie. She seemed to be everywhere, to be spreading herself, and now she'd begun to harass Olwyn. And yet . . . and yet . . . Oliver had shown such skill and maturity in dealing with Mrs Ainsworth who was restored to her normal self, as was Mrs Cider, now back to reading the Bible. Why should he bungle with Coralie?

Mr Albert Cuttle was next. There are obsessionals and obsessionals – and Mr Cuttle, I thought. Obsessional patients are perfectionists, the salt of the earth in many ways. It's only when their industrious and critical natures become exaggerated enough in the form of crippling and anxious rituals and habits (often associated with washing and cleanliness), that they become neurotic and a slave to their obsessions.

Mr Cuttle, a retired bank manager, spent his day racing

around the house washing and rinsing and sending things to the cleaner. He once told me pathetically that his obsession-ality was so bad that he even washed the soap before using it to wash other things! And the medication he took provided more cause for worry. Did it matter whether he took the tablets with water? Before meals? Ground up the medicine? What side effects could he get? Could he drive? And yet if he tried to stop the drugs, as he often had, then his washing and cleaning rituals became totally unbearable.

'I read about these peacemaker things for people with bad hearts. Could I have one? In my brain? I wouldn't mind the operation, if I thought it'd help.'

I must have goggled at him vaguely because he repeated what he'd said rather reproachfully. No, I told him that fitting a 'peacemaker' wouldn't do anything for him. Then couldn't I change his tablets? Try other ones?

We'd been through all this before, many times and I must have sounded a bit sour when I said this, judging by the way poor Mr Cuttle looked at me. I was sorry for being snappy, I said, but I was worried about a patient. Mr Cuttle, making me feel more ashamed, said he quite understood and he was sorry for taking up my time. I was going to explain further and say no, of course not, he wasn't taking up my time at all when the phone rang and Mr Cuttle left.

'Olwyn here, Joyce, I'm afraid Sheena's slipped into what looks like a hypoglycaemic coma. I thought she was just sleeping . . .'

'Oh God,' I said. 'Oliver hasn't arrived here yet. Any chance of getting him over from the hospital?'

'He's on his way here. And I've asked him to bring some glucose because . . .'

'She won't be able to drink so he'll have to get into a vein, and in Sheena's collapsed state that's going to be difficult.'

'Oliver's a whiz on veins, though I say it myself. No, don't worry. I hear Oliver coming . . .'

Damn and double damn! I should have checked Sheena's

blood sugar knowing that stress and lack of food would play hell with her diabetes. Her urine test hadn't been too bad when I'd done it each morning, but the drop in her blood sugar, which showed itself by coma, I should have allowed for.

I must have shown all the worry and distraction I was feeling because the Marsden twins who came in next looked at me askance and hurriedly I said I was recovering from flu.

Di and Mabs Marsden were twins in their seventies who lived and spoke as one although Di, distinguishable by the mole on her chin, was subject to bouts of depression which fortunately could be kept at bay by taking a drug called Lithium three times a day. The blood level was kept regular by periodic blood checks and as Di, who like her sister was a retired teacher, was a most co-operative patient, her equilibrium was maintained and she'd had no more depression since starting the Lithium six years ago. I always rather enjoyed seeing them because they were an Elsie and Doris Waters pair who used all the slang of the 'forties, when they were fire-watchers during the war. I gathered that peace had been an anti-climax. They'd been engaged to two RAF men who'd been shot down over Germany and they'd never had the need to make other relationships. I always thought that the aftermath of the war made them feel so let down that they'd rather settle for peace and each other's company. They even looked like the 'forties with their crimped hair, dark lip-stick and severe suits.

'You're feeling ever so well Di, aren't you, dear?'

'Bang on. I don't know what to do with all my energy. But I have a go, don't I, Mabs?'

'She's even wanting to start a French course on the Open University. What with our yoga, the flower arrangement course and helping with the illiterates at the Education College we're jolly busy.'

False teeth flashing and bellows of laughter from the two

of them. They never changed, ever since I'd known them except when Di had had her depression, and I'd almost forgotten that except that she had used some very bad language indeed!

'I say you're looking a bit tired, Doctor. Isn't she looking tired, Mabs?'

'Excuse us being personal but you are looking . . . well . . . not quite the thing. She's not quite the thing is she, Mabs?'

Like concerned camels they were, the way they peered and preened. What a malicious beast I was. I was very ashamed at my thought because it was nice of my patients to notice me and my appearance.

'Mustn't overdo things, dear. We're none of us getting any younger, are we, Di?'

'As they say, time marches on. Well, we mustn't tire you, dear. Must keep showing the flag, I expect that's your motto as well as ours, Doctor. Toodle-pip then, dear.'

They clattered out and another patient came in.

I thought Oliver would never show up, though when I phoned the house Olwyn said that he'd got some glucose into a vein and Sheena was now round and drinking.

It was after four o'clock when Oliver rushed in, his dark hair flying and his tie crooked. 'She's O.K. Didn't have to have more than twenty cc's of glucose. I've adjusted her insulin and she's promised to eat.'

'Great. I really am so very grateful to you both. I don't know how I'd have managed. Frankie's there of course, but she's always out on calls at this time of the day, and then she has home commitments. It was very smart of Olwyn spotting the coma . . .'

'She's a nurse, you know. And a good one. But she prefers office hours, being off-duty at nights and weekends. Well, I'd better get cracking. There's a mob out there. Ol says you're not to worry, she's staying with Sheena.'

'Is there any news?' I knew the answer to that one.

'I'm afraid not. God, it's such a damnable thing to

happen. About the worst there is. And for a vulnerable girl like Sheena.'

'I know,' I said.

In a way I was glad of the work because it filled the hours, stopping the necessity of staring at a silent phone and having to look at Sheena's pinched misery. But I would have to release Olwyn tomorrow. She had her own life. Her own job.

The patients must have tried to help me by not lingering too long because I was actually through my list by five o'clock. I was ready to leave for home when the phone rang. It was Kate Pillsworth.

'They told me you were doing domiciliary calls, Doctor Delaney.'

'That's right. Urgent calls.' I hoped she'd take the hint that her call had better be a serious one.

'I think the matter is urgent, Doctor Delaney. I think the GP is being . . . well . . . I don't like to say it, but he's a bit dilatory about doing anything to help.'

Such as? Doing what?' Damn the girl, her carping tone was maddening me already.

'Well. It's this old couple, the Laceys, they're both in their seventies and I think they're in grave danger of harming themselves. Setting light to the house or starving themselves.'

'Miss Pillsworth,' I said, 'if the couple are old how is the matter urgent? Presumably things haven't got like this overnight?'

'Well, that's just it you see. I've been on to Doctor Miller, the GP, for ages now but nothing's happened.'

I knew James Miller. He was a tubby little man of immense charm whose heart was so big and kind that he never bothered with appointments but gave, as he put it, a 'Come all ye faithful' service which his patients appreciated so much that they resisted moving out of the area because they were so fond of him.

'Oh, I'm not saying Doctor Miller's wrong,' Kate burbled

on. 'He's very kind and probably thinks he's doing the best thing for the old couple. He couldn't see my point of view when I told him there was so much that we could do to help the Laceys.'

'Miss Pillsworth,' I said, 'have the old couple asked for help?'

'How can they when they don't know what help is available? I mean, there's the meals on wheels, the home help service, the health visitor, the tuck-in service.'

'What,' I asked, 'is the tuck-in service?'

'That's it, you see, people don't know of their entitlements. The tuck-in service is a group of women who go to old folk at risk and living on their own, and they settle them down for the night.'

'Pardon my ignorance,' I said rather coldly. Miss Pillsworth's heavily born knowledge was giving me the usual irritation. I told her I'd be along to Padgate Crescent where the old couple lived within half an hour. She said she'd be waiting for me.

I phoned Olwyn and discovered that Sheena was still sleeping but had eaten some toast. I was just about to leave the clinic room when an enraged Doctor Miller phoned me.

'Has that woman from Social Services phoned you about the Laceys, Doctor Delaney?'

I said she had and I was about to go and see the old couple.

'A rather dirty old pair who are perfectly happy to live, and die, in their own brand of dirt. Now this Pillsworth woman is on the rampage saying nothing's been done, and if she keeps on like this the bloody press'll get hold of it and make something out of it. I've heard about this bitch before, she's succeeded in having a run-in with most of the local doctors.'

He didn't have to tell me anything about the Pillsworth Syndrome, I said.

'She needs some psychiatric treatment herself. Or a big

hairy sailor,' Miller barked. 'Seriously though, I get on with Social Services on the whole, though at times I think they interfere too much. Come between the doctor-patient relationship. We didn't appreciate the days, Doctor Delaney, when you were allowed to get on and treat a patient without people like social workers telling you how to do it, and then skipping out of the way when there's any dirty work like an inquest. But the other social workers are paragons compared to Pillsworth. I apologise for lumbering you with this one but I want to make it clear that it's Miss Pillsworth who's making the fuss, not me. Not only is she sticking her nose into what I regard as my business but she's going around bleating that I'm negligent.'

'I never thought that, James,' I said. 'And I know very well the request isn't from you, but from her.'

'Which is putting the cart before the horse.'

He was to think nothing of it. I'd go out and see the Laceys otherwise Miss Pillsworth would continue bothering people.

'Roll on retirement,' Miller groaned. 'Here's this poor old couple troubling no one and they're not allowed to smell if they want to and live on fish and chips eaten at an open fire.'

I was half-way to the Lacey's house when I remembered that I hadn't spoken to Oliver about Coralie. It would have to keep. Maybe that small inner nagging that there was going to be trouble about her was just a nothing.

Chapter Nine

Number twelve Padgate Crescent was a tumbledown little house tucked away at the end of a wildly overgrown path; so thick and dense was the uncared-for tangle of green clumped on the broken surface, that I nearly tripped several times. The extent of the foliage and the crooked appearance of the stone cottage reminded me of Hansel and Gretel. Especially when I tried to get in. There was a notice written in a straggling print saying 'Go round the back. Bell not working'; and another faded card read 'No Plimuth Bretern'. I noticed the shattered glass of the dusty window and the amount of rusty tin cans in the back garden, which was even more wildly overgrown than the front.

'I've told them Doctor Miller sent you,' Miss Pillsworth muttered when she answered my bang on the back door. 'Look at this kitchen. You see what I mean?'

Yes, by only the most charitable could the dark, smelly little room be called anything as grand as a 'kitchen'. Only the blackened old gas stove and the bulging food cupboard, which was stacked with half opened tins and sagging bags of sugar and flour, bore any relation to the preparation of food. A mangy cat reared up angrily from the kitchen table where it was demolishing some cat food on a saucer.

'The smell. They never clean or wash up anything.'

Miss Pillsworth pointed to the sink which was built like a horse trough and crammed with dirty plates and dishes. Kate Pillsworth shuddered as she nearly slipped on a piece of kipper on the floor. 'I don't know how they survive,' she said.

She was wearing a pink dress which did nothing for her face, now red with anger and heat, and the clumping, flat-heeled sandals cruelly emphasised the lack of shape in her sturdy legs. What with her gingery hair and the shade of her crimplene dress, she reminded me of a fire engine. There was the same amount of energy and steam.

The home help had refused to come until the Public Health Authorities cleansed and fumigated the place, Kate continued, and her own department, Social Services, were fed up with getting their forms returned with Mr Fred Lacey's irreverent scrawls of 'rubbish' on them. Nothing really could be done to help the Laceys of course, till they came into hospital.

'Do you mean Barrington?' I asked.

'Certainly,' replied Miss Pillsworth, hastily lifting her hand from where she'd let it drop into a small puddle of broken egg on the table.

But what if the old couple didn't want to come in? What if they were happy as they were, as their own GP, Doctor Miller, said they were?

That wasn't really the point, was it, Kate said smugly. The Laceys didn't know what was best for them and their welfare. It would be nice of course if they agreed to come in. She had put it to them several times during her frequent visits. Had tried to coax and cajole them, reason and argue with them, told them that a few weeks in Barrington would benefit them and allow people to clean and renovate their home but no, the obstinate pair firmly declined the offer of being made whiter than white. Apart from them having no insight at all, Kate went on, they were a worry to their neighbours and a danger to themselves. They turned up the gas haphazardly, wandered in the garden in their nightgowns, and had a habit of turning up the TV so that it could be heard on the road.

I could have said that people had rights to be nuisances if they so wished. To let down the public weal. The fact that the Laceys were old and messy, and affronted others by their smelly existence wasn't enough to contemplate packing them into a mental hospital. I was tired and cross and the worry about Sheena made my heart a stone. I was afraid to say anything in case I let rip on Kate Pillsworth and said things I'd be sorry for later. Her bossy, prissy manner and the way she strode around like a super-nanny knowing what was best for the children! Tuck-in service, indeed. Miller was right, Miss Pillsworth needed some attention herself. all that ferocious energy which should have come out in a sexual way was being sublimated and canalised into her work, and used to fire the awesome inner-batteries. Of course, she'd been correct about Mr Dippy. She'd sounded off about the care and thought that should be put into the matter of committing people to a psychiatric hospital. Here she was now doing a volte face about the Laceys. What an unpredictable girl she was. Still, I thought, I must control myself, mustn't let myself get goaded by Miss Pillsworth into overreacting. Especially without seeing the old folk.

'Mr Lacey, Fred, is a bit deaf so that's why they have the TV so loud.'

Miss Pillsworth rushed over to the enormous set which looked as if it might topple at any minute from the ramshackle table it was perched on. This room was as bad as the kitchen. The pokey little windows could have been boarded up for all the light they gave, and no wonder the old pair had the ceiling light on, though it was only seven o'clock on a bright summer's evening. While Kate twiddled with knobs and only increased the roar of the Mohican braves as they fell upon the snaking procession of white settlers who made a bursting return of guns, the old couple heaved themselves up from roasting their skinny shins at the coal fire.

'That's another thing. Their fuel bills are astronomical because they use the fire even in a heatwave,' Kate hissed, over the roar of the TV which she at last managed to turn off.

''Ere, Miss Pillsworth. I was watching that Western. I

love it when they start the fighting.' The old man who spoke was dressed in a grey, tattered vest and his raggedy pants gaped to show his withered privates.

'Yes, he sometimes 'ops into bed and watches from there,' Mrs Lacey smiled toothlessly and then rummaged in her bag, found her false teeth and rammed them in. Either her gums had shrunk or she's put them in wrong, because they made her face lop-sided. She wore a stained, old satin dressing-gown which she pulled against her concave chest with a veiny hand. She nearly bald, with some fine, white fuzz erupting here and there on her pate.

'I've brought a lady doctor to see you. Doctor Miller sent her. She may be able to help you,' Kate said.

Mr Lacey belched and said crossly, 'Then he 'adn't ought to. We're all right, 'ilda and me. Ain't we, love?'

'Happy as two bugs. We've been married sixty years Fred and me come August next.'

Kate drew away from the motheaten poodle which suddenly appeared. After getting the brush-off from Miss Pillsworth the little dog jumped on to Mrs Lacey's lap.

'She's got fleas, that dog,' Kate whispered and then out loud she told the Laceys that they needed looking after, their family was too far away, and they were no longer able to cope with living on their own.

'I'm not going in no 'ome,' Fred shouted, pushing his face forwards so that his stringy neck made him look like an enraged turtle.

'We're all right 'ere, duck. Just 'im and me. We're warm, we eats what we likes and we get up when we likes . . .'

That was the whole point, Kate Pillsworth said. She had a very annoying habit of shaking her finger at people, like a teacher at dull pupils. What had the pair eaten today?

'Well. We 'ad dripping toast in the morning and then, come three o'clock, we made us some fried onions and carrots,' Fred Lacey said.

I butted in when Kate started on about the couple's lack

of balanced meals, and said that they were both healthy looking which indeed they were. They may have been shabby and rather dirty, but their eyes were bright and their skin, such as could be seen under the coating of dirt, was not showing any evidence of starvation.

'We eats what we wants, when we wants and Doctor Miller, he comes once a week, more if we want 'im, and he gives us the once-over like, and he says we're all right. We never been in no hospital either of us for forty years and we ain't a-goin' in now. So you can go back to Doc Miller and tell him to stick that in his pipe.'

Poor Mr Lacey's face crumpled and his wife's eyes filled with tears. I suddenly couldn't stand the hectoring bullying of Miss Pillsworth a moment longer, but before I could rally my raging thoughts Fred started again.

'You go into them places you never come out,' Fred began to scratch himself and Mrs Lacey flapped her old hands distractedly.

'We don't want nothing done here. The place will see us out. We didn't ask for help cause we're so happy here. We don't want no Boy Scouts doing the garden or women coming in and out interfering with the way we live. We just want to be left alone till they come with the coffins for us.' She patted the dingy poodle fiercely and went on, 'It's Barrington Hall, the Workhouse . . . that's where they want to put us . . .'

Nothing like that, Kate Pillsworth explained. They'd come home after a rest and feel much better able to live the wholesome life which they were entitled to.

'There's such a thing as quality of life,' she said and really I thought, with her earnest, preaching manner, she's missed her vocation.

There was no need to be frightened, I told the Laceys, I certainly wouldn't recommend that they be moved and neither would Doctor Miller. Kate Pillsworth looked at me as if I was a black traitor.

'I don't know why Doctor Miller thought as we wanted Barrington . . .' Fred said puzzled.

Poor old things, I thought, this will upset and worry them for ages, the fear that intrusive busy-bodies like Kate would walk into their home and threaten a sort of eviction. I'd contact Doctor Miller, I said, and tell him what I was telling them.

It was as if I'd pulled a gun on Kate. She shook her red hair and asked what did I mean? Surely I saw that the Laceys would do something to themselves, set fire to the house or be found dead from hypothermia and malnutrition?

Let's wait till that happens, I said, and take it from there. They were not demented, they weren't doing anything illegal, and if they were more intelligent and aggressive they might well bring a case for harassment against Social Services.

Kate boggled. Here she was doing everything that the government pamphlet 'Care of the Aged' advised and here was *me* levelling harassment at her. Didn't I realise she was only trying to apply the spirit of the modern code of Community Care to the Laceys?

'But you're tackling it the wrong way, Miss Pillsworth,' I said. 'Instead of working to make the community accept the Laceys, dirt and warts and all, you are trying to force an old couple to change *their* ways to fit the *community* and that is just cruel and stupid.'

Her face wobbled and she paled, staring almost wildly, as if I had dealt her some mortal blow in her most sensitive part. 'But I'm only doing my job. What if something happens? I mean, I am only trying to help, Doctor. And the way I see my function –'

'That's the trouble, Miss Pillsworth. The way you see your job is not the correct way, not the most humane or compassionate way. You are a self-opinionated, bossy woman who has succeeded in clashing with the GPs, telling them how to do their job, and they're too gentlemenly to tell you to go to hell. But I'm not a gentleman and I'm sick and tired of you and your messing –' She opened her mouth but nothing came so I shouted, 'And don't point your finger at me! I'm not one of your "clients", thank God.'

I was so mad I don't know how I hadn't an accident on the way home and my last sight of Miss Pillsworth was seeing her in my car mirror standing, sagging almost, with a stupefied expression on her face. She'd report me to the Director of Social Services I was sure. And probably I'd be black-listed by all her colleagues. To hell with it, I didn't feel good but I didn't regret anything about my attack. The cruel intrusion into the Lacey's lives made me crawl inside. It was like taking sweets from blind children.

I must have shown my anger because Olwyn looked at me apprehensively when I came in. 'Just a run in with a female who shouldn't even do veterinary, leave alone social work,' I said.

Olwyn looked at me compassionately as I sat down wearily. I wasn't tired from the day's work but the Pillsworth episode had left me drained and exhausted. She was young and inexperienced and anxious to do her job well. That was just the trouble. Enthusiasm wasn't enough; the Pillsworth psyche was so blinkered and tactless, and I doubted if she could ever be of real use to patients. But I should have shown more tact myself, yelling at her like an irate market woman. Well, it was done now.

I asked Olwyn about Sheena. Had there been any news?

No news, said Olwyn, bringing in some coffee, but the girl was better in the sense that she was no longer hypoglycaemic and had eaten some toast. But that was because Sheena had no energy or resources to refuse what was brought to her. It was, in a way, easier for her to play along. The will to live was dying in Sheena, Olwyn went on. Melinda had meant a tie to the living, a commitment to hope, for the girl.

'But *I'm* telling you your job,' Olwyn said. 'Oh, that poor,

poor kid. It's not fair. It's just not fair. She had so little and that's been taken away from her.'

I was beginning to be resigned to that myself. It was several days now since Melinda was snatched. And no news. No clues, even. What would happen next? I knew what I thought; any minute now the phone would go and there would be information about a child's body. It would be wrapped up a bit, of course, all the police were family people, but I had seen enough mangled children's bodies to realise what the message meant. A bruised child's corpse on wasteland; or the swollen obscenity of a body dragged from a river or lake; or the end result of a raped small girl, stuffed behind the rubbish in some alley.

I shook off my morbid imaginings as much as I could. But I couldn't, no matter how I tried, shake off the repulsive picture of someone clapping a hand over the screaming Melinda's mouth and the ease with which steady pressure on a small throat could so easily and brutally erase life. Olwyn, I suppose, could see I was very upset. She was a naturally perceptive girl and her nursing experience must stand to her. I didn't feel like eating, the thought of food stuck fast in my throat but it was too much of an effort to refuse Olwyn when she offered to heat up some soup for me. Meanwhile there was Sheena.

She was lying back, her normally shiny hair tied with a black velvet ribbon, and someone, Olwyn probably, had put a clean nightgown on her. The face was tiny and so pale that the eyes burned darkly, big black pools of despair. She couldn't even manage to attempt the smile that she'd sometimes given me before. Just the interrogative, desperate question.

'No news, Sheena,' I said.

'I know in my mind and heart that Melinda's dead,' she said. 'Yet, till things are settled, I mean, when we hear where Melinda's found, I can't stop myself reacting when people come in.'

I sat down on the chair beside her bed. I was rather proud of the spare room. I'd sewed and put up the red-sprigged muslin curtains which matched the duvet cover, and I'd painted all the surfaces with a white gloss paint which justified it's expense. But the hollow-eyed girl in the bed mocked the freshness of her surroundings.

Rather than trot out what could be nothing more than cruel banalities I reached for Sheena's pale hand. It felt like a small, lifeless fish.

Sheena turned her listless face to me. Everyone had been so very, very kind, she said. Mrs Stafford, her husband, and Doctor Mullen had called at lunch time. Then she closed her eyes and groaned. It was harsh and primitive and despairing. Something like a banshee wail that I'd heard of in rural Ireland. And something very like the sounds of terror she'd made when she'd been psychotically ill. 'Why can't the police do something? It's their job, isn't it? Everyone cares but nobody can *do* anything.'

I sat with her till the sedative I gave her sent her into a restless, drowsy state. It was dark when Olwyn called to me from the doorway to say that my soup which had been reheated twice, would be cold if I didn't have it now.

As I sipped tomato soup Olwyn drew the curtains. What about Oliver? I asked. There was no sound from the Staffords' flat below.

'He's on duty and one of the patients sprang an acute abdomen so the theatre had to be opened, there was no time to send the patient to St Basil's. One of the surgeons came out though, and Oliver's assisting. But that's what he likes,' she added, 'the more work the better.'

As I drank the soup, which slipped down more easily than I'd thought would be possible, I pondered about Olwyn. Was there a touch of bitterness in the way she'd talked about Oliver's penchant for work? The first impressions of her, that she was a rather naïve, provincial girl, basking in the reflected glory of her husband, couldn't be more wrong.

Naïve she wasn't, in spite of that soft accent and her beauty which was so dazzling it was almost a distracting red herring from her very real intelligence. Tonight, and probably because of Sheena, she looked worn and in spite of the poor light, I noticed the tracks of small lines at the sides of her violet eyes. There was even a deep line etched between each side of her nose and mouth. She was older than I'd thought. Older looking than Oliver, whose fly-away clothes and untidy mop of hair gave him a juvenile, distrait appearance. I'd guess he hadn't changed much in appearance and manner from when he was a student. Now that he'd gained some weight and acquired a tan, which had lifted his former dead-white pallor, his Byronic good looks were more evident.

'She talked to me quite a lot this afternoon. Said that she hadn't wanted to come out of the coma,' said Olwyn. 'And I did my best to comfort her. Not to take all hope away.'

I was sure she did her best I said. After all, the two girls couldn't be far removed in age.

'But when she heard I didn't have children I'm afraid I lost credibility for her. She was too nice to say what I'm sure she was feeling, that I am a selfish woman, well able to provide a home for a baby.'

'I'm sure Sheena wasn't thinking like that, Olwyn. She's been through too much not to realise that things, or people, aren't what they seem, and that the reasons for having or not having babies aren't simple.'

'That's the nice explanation, the charitable one,' Olwyn said, and now there was real bitterness in her tone as she put dishes on the tray.

Something wrong with that area of her life. It would explain Oliver's lack of ambition or maybe, as Olwyn herself had confided to me before, the reason for his not having settled. But I was tired in an aching, bone weary way. I'd had enough emotion to last me for weeks and my row with Kate Pillsworth had upset me.

Go to bed, Olwyn begged me, she'd clear up and sit for a while till Oliver came back. And I was to stay put in the morning, he'd see to things. But there was my clinic at St Basil's, in the afternoon. To cancel or send a stand-in to a clinic meant administrative muddle and patients didn't like it. No, I'd have to do my clinic, I told Olwyn, who said that in that case she'd stay with Sheena. When I expressed thanks and doubt about how she'd manage her own job, she said that the partners were most concerned about Sheena and had told Olwyn that of course she must stay with Sheena.

'They are all terribly kind in the firm,' Olwyn said. 'The senior partner is very involved with the Samaritans you know.'

And I had a lot of time for the Samaritans, I said. Many of my patients owed their lives to being able to talk to a Samaritan at three o'clock in the morning.

On the way to bed I decided to phone the police just to hear whether there had been any sort of clue at all. I was, like Sheena, becoming convinced that any news must by now, be that of finding a dead child's body.

'I'm afraid we've had nothing in so far, Doctor.' PC Wiggin was off-duty but the young policeman in his place was solicitous, real concern tempering the official words. They, the police, had chased up all known pederasts, interviewed hundreds of 'contacts'.

'And tomorrow we're going to start dredging the rivers and ponds and that . . .' The policeman was anxious to show me that the Force were being thorough but his words struck a chill. That was it then. They were down to looking for a dead, not a living child.

Tired as I was, the confirmation of my worst fears for Melinda kept sleep away, especially as the welcome rain had gone and the July night was as torrid as the tropics. I tossed and turned and sleep only came at half past five, and was then so stuporous that I didn't hear Olwyn coming in with coffee until the phone shrilled beside me and Olwyn said that it was Doctor Mullen. She'd phoned at eight o'clock and said she'd ring back at nine.

'Didn't know it was so late,' I said and then added, 'there's no news. The police say they're trying the rivers and ponds and things today. It's bad, Frankie.'

'Looks like it. Very black. I was sorry I couldn't be more helpful about Sheena's hypoglycaemia but I was very tied up. There's a dysentery outbreak and it's playing hell with all the babies. Look, about Saturday night . . . the day after tomorrow, I think we'd better scrub it, don't you?'

I'd forgotten all about the proposed meal for the Staffords and me. Yes, it was out, quite definitely, I said. And then something strained about her tone of voice made me wonder. Was she all right? And Barney? I was so het up about Sheena that other people's needs seemed remote.

'Not so well. A gastric upset. Could be dysentery, only Barney's tummy seems to have taken over from his chest. You know what he's like,' Frankie said, 'throwing his hearing aid around the room, breaking thermometers and bellowing his opinion of doctors. Won't see Harper, of course. He's had indigestion for some time and insists on treating himself with mixtures he buys from the chemist. It's no use talking to him. He says he knows as much about dysentery as any quack because it was endemic in India.'

Voltaire would have loved Barney, I thought, as I sipped my coffee.

The morning crawled by. I was ashamed of the relief I felt at getting out to my clinic. Sheena's poor ravaged eyes reproached me. Olwyn and I had managed to get her to have a bath and dress. Even in the space of a few days she'd lost so much weight that her dress sagged on her and her legs were like sticks. When the phone rang at midday she jumped convulsively and turned ashen. God! My God! The police had found Melinda in the canal, I thought. I jumped myself when I heard who was calling.

'It's Kate Pillsworth here, Doctor.'

I braced myself for the well-known irritation, the accusations that I had been rude and aggressive and personally abusive. Well, I was damned if I was going to apologise or retract what I'd said. Maybe the way I'd said it had been wrong but I still thought she was high-handed and tactless. She needn't think I was going to whitewash one atom of what I had said about the poor old Laceys. But she proceeded to take every puff of wind out of my sails.

She was terribly sorry, she said abjectly. I was right to take her to task. Would I give her another chance? It wasn't the first time she'd been complained about to the Director of Social Services and she was certain that he would transfer her to another department at the very least, indeed, she might be dismissed.

'I've been too busy with another very serious matter to get down to writing about you, Miss Pillsworth,' I said. I was appeased by her admission. And having spoken about not giving up hope on Sheena maybe I ought not to give up on Kate. After all, she was capable of kindness; there was her concern for Mr Dippy, and I was sure she was motivated well. The trouble was her *attitude* which was high-handed and lacking in the crudest form of tact.

She realised it, she said meekly. She would try and improve.

'I'll overlook it on this occasion,' I told her, 'on one condition; that you keep away from the Laceys and apologise to Doctor Miller.'

Oh yes, yes, she said, and was about to repeat her own regret about her behaviour when I cut her short saying I wanted the lines kept clear.

Later, on the way to the clinic, I wondered whether I'd been wise not to cash in on this latest example of Kate's messing and let events take their course, especially as the girl herself was admitting she'd been wrong. It was a golden opportunity to get rid of her. But then, in view of her apology, wasn't she due a last chance to change her ways? I suspected that the Pillsworth personality was beyond change, but enthusiastic workers weren't all that common and Kate was activated by zeal even though that zeal was misdirected. Anyway, I was too busy to do anything at the moment so I decided to give her the benefit of proving herself.

When I got to St Basil's I found I was a bit early, although Oliver had started work, the young nurse told me. From the corner of my eye I could see Coralie, dressed in sugar pink, chatting to one of my patients. It was Alan Moore, a young psychopath, who specialised in dabbling with LSD, sniffing glue, and making himself a nuisance to every hospital by turning up in a state of collapse from alcohol and drugs and conning the young housemen who admitted him. He was staring down into Coralie's cleavage and maybe it was because I was worried, tired and depressed, but I suddenly got furious about the presence of two time-wasters like Coralie Kane and Moore. I'd put the skids on him before and said I wouldn't see him again and yet here he was turning up at my clinic full of whining self pity, striking up an acquaintance with that arch manipulator Mrs Kane. Why was she attending the clinic so much? What on earth was Oliver playing at? I thought, as Sister came bustling in. I must have looked bad because Stafford and Sister looked at me with concern.

'No more news, Joyce?' Oliver asked.

'No. Except that they're beginning to try the canals and those sort of places.' The room was hotter than ever and when I sat down the cheap plastic of the chair was burning. 'Any chance of a fan, Sister?' I sounded the way I felt, edgy.

Poor Sister jumped up saying how sorry she was, she should have remembered I liked the small table fan in this weather.

'Oliver,' I said, 'how are you are you getting on with Mrs Kane? Only she seems to be coming a lot.'

Oliver shifted in his chair. He needed a hair cut and for all Olwyn's attempts to get him to take more care with his clothes, his shirt was creased and, really, he should give that old dark suit away. It hung on his body in baggy folds.

'Oh . . . I'm continuing her psychotherapy. I see her every week and it seems to be benefiting her. I think she's probably better with a male therapist, you know.'

'I hope you know what you're doing, Oliver. Mrs Kane has a nasty habit of compromising men. She's had a go at involving her dentist, a social worker and a probation officer.'

'For what?' Oliver looked at me warily.

'For "making advances" as it's called. She eats up men Doesn't like them, I suspect, and tries to destroy them.'

Oliver smiled and said mildly that he thought he could manage. Mrs Kane had high defences and was rather paranoid but he thought he could manage. He was so magnanimous and mild that I was now angry at my own ill-temper. Besides, here he was doing my work and Olwyn was sitting minding Sheena. I was a small-minded, petty bitch, I thought, as Sister reappeared with the fan which she plugged in. Oliver further added to my contrition when he said I mustn't worry. He knew what he was doing. I said I was sorry and it was due to my fears for Sheena. He smiled at me and said that I was to be sure and let him know when I wanted to go. He'd manage.

'Charming fellow,' Morgan said, puce and panting after her exertions on my behalf. 'The patients adore him. Nothing's too much trouble for him. Listens for hours and gets right through to them, even Mrs Kane. He's got endless patience with her.'

Coals of fire. Coals of fire, I thought, and told Sister I was sorry for being snappy, it was because I was so worried about Sheena Boden.

'I've got something to tell you, Doctor. It may be something or nothing and maybe I'm an old busy body but I thought you ought to know. My friend, Sister Madigan, works in the Maternity and she told me yesterday that she was reading about the Boden child and remembered that one of your patients had been seen staring at the babies. She had to be told to leave and got very upset. Madigan said that she was a very thin, plain-looking girl who had a mad, sort of vacant look about her and that she, Maddy, was afraid that the girl might be tempted to steal a child. That's when she heard the girl was Wendy Cotton, a patient of yours, and that her trouble is sterility. I just thought there might be some connection, some tie-up with this poor girl who's had her child taken . . .'

Wendy Cotton? Wendy Cotton. I didn't even jabber a 'thank you' to Morgan, but raced off to ask Oliver to take over for me. I didn't know when I'd be back.

I thought of that hungry longing on Mrs Cotton's eyes. Could she have taken Melinda?

Chapter Ten

I had to talk to someone. I sat and waited till Oliver was finished, which meant another hour and a half because he always took longer than me. I asked Sister to tell him that I wanted to see him urgently and began turning things over and over in my mind. What had to be done was to call on Wendy. Her craving for a child and her appearance in the Maternity Unit might be all coincidental, but then again maybe it meant something. She wasn't bright, certainly much less intelligent than Sheena, but surely even Wendy Cotton didn't think she'd get away with stealing another woman's child? That's if Mrs Cotton were in a normal state of mind. Which she wasn't. Cases of baby snatching were not unknown in women whose babies had died, and Wendy's plight was worse than having a dead baby really, for there was no hope of another child.

'Wow.' Oliver said when I told him. 'Something or nothing, this bit of news. Let's go and see Wendy now.'

'You'll come with me?'

'Sure. No bother. Let's go.'

A soft, misty summer shower had cooled the dusty air and we drove to Wendy's house. The wheels hissed on the wet road and Oliver stared out of the window, arms folded.

'I went back to help in Aberfan, you know. We all did from the neighbouring villages. Some of the kids were unmarked, just as if they were asleep. You picked them up and they were like little dolls, sort of limp.'

Wendy's house was deserted but the curtains weren't drawn and there were no empty milk bottles. I rang the bell a few times but there was no answer, no sign of life at all, much less any signs of a child. While Oliver went around to the back I walked down the path to the road. A large woman in a red pixie hood and plastic mac smiled at me.

'Looking for Mrs Cotton are you?'

I said yes, but there was no answer when we'd pressed the bell.

'Funny, I live next door and I haven't seen Wendy this week. Usually see her twice a week at the supermarket. Mind you, she suffers with her nerves and I know she's under the doctor. Are you from the Welfare?'

'No,' I replied. People were always asking me whether I was from the Welfare!

'Sorry I can't tell you nothing, Wendy's a quiet little thing, ever so quiet and she keeps herself to herself. Her husband's on nights now, of course, maybe that has something to do with it. Night shifts don't give you no real rest, not when you got to sleep during the days in summer.'

As the woman went away Oliver appeared and waved for me to come and try again. I pressed the bell really hard and this time there was the sound of someone coming downstairs and then the door opened and Wendy appeared.

'Was you ringing long? I was having me bath.'

That was true, her hair was hanging in a wet and raggedy fringe and there was a reek of violet bath salts from her. She seemed to be taking more of an interest in her appearance, no matter how unfortunate the results. I hadn't seen the mauve dress before and I'd never seen her wear lipstick, but now her mouth was garishly outlined in crimson.

'What's the matter? Why have you come?' She looked like a hare blinded by car lights and kept shooting glances at Oliver. She obviously wasn't going to ask us to come in.

'Well. The thing is that I heard you'd been seen in the Maternity Unit at St Chad's and I wondered whether you were all right, Wendy.'

Too bald, too challenging, I realised, as soon as I'd said it. I should have been less outspoken, wrapped things up a bit more. But my thoughts were with the wretched Sheena.

'How did you hear? I didn't do nothin' wrong, did I?' She sounded frenzied and I felt like a heel.

'I wondered whether you were all right. I know how terrible you felt about not having a child of your own.'

'I was only looking. There isn't any signs up to say you can't have a look. I suppose that snooty nurse who asked me who I was went and told you, didn't she?'

There wasn't much I could do about the next question. It had to be asked. I had to know, if only for poor Sheena's sake. 'Wendy,' I said, 'I've got to ask you something. And please be honest . . .' She shook the damp fringe from her eyes and pushed the hair back with a small claw hand which was tipped plum red. Her glance flicked from Oliver to me. Hunted. Two against one. In spite of my worry about Melinda I was stabbed with pity for this poor girl. No more than for Sheena, nothing seemed to have gone right for Wendy, nothing at all, and here we were, as she thought, to persecute her again. 'Somebody I know, a girl about your age, well, her three-year-old child's gone missing and I wondered whether you knew anything about it?'

She paled and grabbed at the side of the door as if she had to support herself. 'I don't know what you're talking about. Coming like this, asking me questions, accusing me . . .' Her voice trailed off despairingly and I felt ashamed. Bad enough to be sterile without having people coming to probe you about baby snatching. I tried again.

'This girl, the mother, is very ill. If the child isn't found soon the mother may die. Please, Wendy, tell me if you know anything about it.'

'I told you. I told you. I don't know nothin'. You come here harassing me. You're supposed to help people, you are, but oh, no, you come around when me husband's at work asking me questions, sticking your nose into my business when I 'aven't done nothing to no one.' She burst into loud sobs, choking and gasping like a child with convulsions.

'So you don't know anything about the child, Wendy? That's true?'

She smeared a hand across her teary face. 'I told you didn't I?'

'Because I have to go back and tell the mother, Wendy, tell her that there's no news about the child.'

'I don't care what you tell her. That's your look out isn't it? Anyway, anyway, she can have another kid can't she?'

Wendy shouted the last as she slammed the door and I turned to Oliver. He hadn't been much help but then perhaps he thought I wanted to deal with things. And I hadn't. Hadn't been tactful at all, I told him as we went down the path.

'Hard to be diplomatic about asking Wendy whether she whipped the kid,' he said. 'No way of getting around it really.'

'What do you think?' I asked him as we drove home. 'I can't believe she's telling us the truth.'

He didn't answer and seemed to be slumped in a day dream. Just when I could have done with a bit of help, I thought crossly. Well, it was a good thing I hadn't said anything to Sheena about suspecting Wendy.

'Can you tell me what the kid was wearing?' Oliver asked.

Yes, I'd had to tell that to the police. Melinda had been wearing a pale blue dress, white socks and dark blue shoes. Why had he asked?

'Nothing really,' he said and lapsed into silence again. Well, it was after seven o'clock and maybe he was tired. Even his energy must have limits. I was surprised then when, after we'd pulled up in front of the Priest's House, he said he had to go back to the hospital about something, and drove off through the heavy and persistent rain.

Olwyn opened my front door for me.

'Sheena's sleeping, flat out she is. Look, you look exhausted, would you like me to fetch you some food? I have a steak and kidney pie and . . .'

'No thanks Olwyn. Maybe I'll feel like it later, though. Oliver dashed back to the hospital.'

Olwyn shrugged and said that that figured. I was to let her know if there was any news. I noticed she hadn't asked me, probably could tell by my face that there was nothing.

After I'd made some tea I looked in on Sheena who was laying motionless on her side, and for a terrible moment I thought she was dead, she breathed so quietly. I was coward enough to be glad she wasn't awake and that I didn't have to face the question in her sick eyes. There were things I ought to do, my food was running low and I had several bills to pay. Which reminded me that I needed money from the bank. Life went on after all; I'd have to find some time soon to do some shopping. I had got as far as making a list when the phone rang.

'Any idea when Oliver is returning?' Olwyn wanted to know. 'I tried the hospital and he's not there. In fact, he seems not to have been there since this morning. You said he'd gone there.'

Funny, I'd distinctly heard him say he was going. Some of the wards didn't have good telephone lines, I told her, and it was always possible that his bleep wasn't working and that he could still be in the hospital.

'Yes. Oh, well, he'll just have to eat frizzled pie,' she said.

I had just got back to my chair when the phone rang again; it was Oliver.

'Now listen, Joyce,' he said. 'I've got Melinda and she's all right. Wendy had her. Kept her in a shed in the garden.'

'Oh, my God! But that's tremendous. So that's where you went. Well done. But how did you know she was there, Oliver?'

'Noticed a blue shoe on the floor in the hall when we were talking to Wendy,' he said.

'This is marvellous news, Oliver. Just marvellous. And Wendy?'

'Pretty shook up. You can imagine. I've told the police

and tried to prop Wendy up by telling her that I think she'll be sent to have some treatment rather than to prison. Anyway her husband's on his way and I'm bringing Melinda back in a taxi.'

I dialled three wrong numbers before my hand was steady enough to get Olwyn, who gave a whoop when she heard the news. Great observation on Oliver's part, I said. And now I must tell Sheena.

She was awake when I went in, lying back on the pillows looking mutely at me. Not even asking me. I guessed her thoughts; she was thinking that her child must be dead.

'It's all right, Sheena,' I said, sitting down on the edge of the bed. How translucent her skin was, papery with the blood vessels standing out like small snakes. 'Melinda is all right. We've found her. Oliver is bringing her now . . . in a taxi.'

Her lips were so cracked and her dry tongue so sore that she had difficulty speaking. She licked her caked lips and asked, 'Where was she? Is she . . .' She had difficulty forming the words. 'Is she all right? Safe? Not hurt?'

She was fine, I said again, and Sheena began to sob hoarsely, dry, rasping sounds which were very painful to hear. I put my arms around her and I don't know how long we sat like that with Sheena just clinging and clutching and me having to repeat several times the news which had been so late in coming. Then I heard the taxi draw up and I helped Sheena to put on her dressing gown and tie back her hair. Oliver appeared holding Melinda and Sheena snatched the child who looked as plump and happy as ever. It was only when poor Sheena in her joy hugged the child too hungrily that Melinda began to cry.

'Where was she? Who took her?' Sheena was weeping, the tears making rivers through her dehydrated skin.

'A patient of mine who couldn't have a child of her own,' I said. 'She'd been seen looking at the babies in the Maternity Unit, so we got suspicious and called to see her this evening but she denied it. Oliver was quick enough to notice one of Melinda's shoes in the hall and he went back.'

'I think she was glad to tell me in the end, you know,' Oliver said. 'Knowing it would be only a matter of time before the kid was discovered.'

'I can never thank you enough, Doctor Stafford, honestly I can't.' Sheena felt her child all over and Melinda started scrambling to get down, crying with tiredness. She'd better put Melinda to bed, Sheena said, and made a gesture at Oliver, trying to say something but not being able to find the right words. Oliver looked embarrassed and said that he was glad everything had turned out all right.

'Just luck I spotted the shoe,' Oliver said and then, as if anticipating more gratitude, he added that Olwyn would be wondering where he was and he'd better go.

I felt like some food and was just wondering whether left-over stew would do, when Sheena appeared. Amazing, I thought, how in less than an hour she was transformed into a happy young girl. Radiant, you could call her.

'Mel's asleep. You know, she has been well cared for. Didn't even want her usual scoff of a chocolate biscuit. I wouldn't want the poor girl who took her to go to prison.'

I didn't think that would happen, I said. I'd guess that Wendy would be made the subject of a court order which ensured treatment. Which she badly needed.

'I'd like to see her sometime later, and help her if I could. I know something about loneliness and being depressed,' Sheena said.

It was always like that, the people who had least to give wanted to give. Maybe Sheena could make Wendy come to terms with her lot. But that would have to wait. Meantime, there were mundane things to think of, like food. Could stew tempt Sheena?

'On one condition,' she said, 'that I heat it up. Please let me. You look whacked, Doctor Delaney. Do have a rest while I make supper.'

'I'd love a bath,' I said.

As I was going out of the room Sheena called me, 'I'd like to go back to my flat tomorrow, Doctor Delaney. If that's all right with you.'

I had a lovely, slow soak and was just about to call to Sheena that she could serve up the stew, when the phone rang and it was Frankie asking if there was anything fresh about Melinda. She gave a joyous yelp when I told her the news and I could make out Barney's roars in the background.

'Smashing. Just smashing,' Frankie shouted. 'You have to hand it to Oliver, noticing the shoe. I bet Sheena's in heaven.'

'She's come back to life,' I told her.

'Listen then,' Frankie continued, 'Saturday night is on. I want you and the Staffords to come over for a meal, sevenish.'

Fine, I said. Sheena was laying the table and I never realised that stew could smell so good. I told Frankie I'd see her on Saturday and was about to put down the phone when I remembered to ask about Barney. Maybe we should postpone visiting till he was better?

'Oh no. Visitors will cheer him up. I think he's caught a bug. Terrific indigestion and he will keep dosing himself with stone-age remedies like magnesia and what he calls "bread soda". Anything I say is suspect, of course, and I can't get him to see Harper. He'll survive though, the Osborne constitution's like a lion's. See you, and best love to Sheena.'

Of course the whole hospital was humming with the news of the restoration of Melinda and of Oliver's part in it. When I went into the canteen for lunch I saw Tony Manners beckoning to me from a free table. I didn't particularly want to join him. I felt tired and draggy this morning. I liked

Manners well enough but I never felt he wanted to talk to people merely for conversation; it was usually with a view to expert pumping and I wasn't in the mood to be pumped. He was one of the new breed of bright young consultant and wore a yellow tie and suede jacket. He had an irritating knack of making me feel passé. I longed for him to make a mistake but he got on with everyone, even with Coulter.

'I hear the Boden kid is safe and sound,' he said. 'Stafford to the rescue?'

Frankie and I had worked out the not too sophisticated psychopathology of Tony Manners. He retained his popularity and the reputation of being the most amiable of the Barrington consultants by an expert knowledge of who was sleeping, having a row or paranoid, with who, and by feeling out the prevailing winds in the hospital he was able to tack and trim his own sails with such precision that he always made harbour. Expert dirt digger that he was, he was adept at giving doses of information on the theory that you had to speculate to accumulate. He was much more shrewd and subtle in his relationships than Coulter, and popular in spite of his gossiping. After all, said Frankie, he was more human then Felix who was only really interested, we thought, in his career and his car.

'Quite the Beloved Doctor our Oliver,' Manners said.

My reaction was to defend Oliver by praising him excessively but I remembered that Manners was powerful as he sat on so many committees and he could be helpful if Oliver wanted a job at Barrington.

'He was the one who spotted a clue about the kid and so was able to get her back quickly. He's an excellent doctor, a real worker. I was wondering, in fact, whether he wouldn't be a candidate for Coulter's job,' I said.

'He's not consultant material,' Manners said acidly. Missed the boat there, all that wandering and nothing to show for it.'

'There's a registrar's job going. Surely he'd be able for that?' I asked.

'We'll see,' Manners said cryptically. 'He seems to be a bit of a womaniser. Not the type of man who's career-minded.'

I was amazed, stopped in my tracks. With a wife as pretty as Olwyn, I was flabbergasted to think of philandering.

'Oh yes,' Manners went on. 'Quite a bit of talk about him hobnobbing with that nurse on Gilbert Ward. Mona Wynn. You know who I mean?'

Sure, I knew Mona, I said. I'd worked with her when she was a student nurse and had been impressed with her interest and ability. She was very good, excellent at her work, I said.

'Oh, she's good at something,' Manners sneered.

Really, he had all the patronising righteousness of the reformed rake. I remembered Manners when he was a senior registrar, before he married when he was having a varied and amorous career. My meat was proving too tough and my conversation with Tony too unproductive, so I jumped up and said I had work to do in Gilbert Ward. I hadn't managed to call there earlier.

On the way out of the canteen I saw Oliver approaching with Mona Wynn. They were immersed in each other, laughing together with a private complicity. Hell, there couldn't, surely there couldn't be anything in Manner's poison?

'Good afternoon.' I didn't think Oliver had seen me but Mona Wynn was quicker and smiled at me. She was small, with rather blunt features but she had an amazing smile and enormous green-yellow eyes. A mass of hair with blonde streaks and that big wide smile. Nothing much when you became specific but the net result was very attractive, electric almost. When Oliver smiled, too, she passed on politely, making for the canteen.

'She's got a Welsh grannie, you know.' Oliver said, staring after her.

He looks so appreciative, I thought. God, I wonder if there is anything in what Manners has been telling me? The thought was so uncomfortable that I smacked it down.

'How's the mother and child this morning?' Oliver asked.

Fine, fine, I said, thanks to him. I was on my way to Gilbert, was there any patient he wanted me to see?

'Not really. I went through most of them this morning. Thought you might take the day off. Oh, Latimer wants a word with you. I don't know what about but he looks dead serious.'

That could mean trouble as Latimer had finely developed nostrils for danger.

When I got to the ward he was waiting for me, sitting at his desk looking serious and solemn. I was just the person he wanted a few words with. He opened the door of the office, peered each way and returned to his seat, one pudgy finger at his mouth. 'We've got a few patients with a nasty habit of lurking at doors,' he said. 'I thought I'd better have words with you, Doctor. It's about Doctor Stafford. Now, I think the world of him. Tip-top at his job. Can't be faulted. And I can't blame him in some ways. Not his fault if he's tempted . . .'

Really, I found Latimer's heavy-handed hints and innuendoes hard to take, tired as I was and still smarting at Manner's remarks. 'What exactly is it, Mr Latimer?' I asked.

'That Nurse Wynn. I never wanted her on the ward. Never really wanted female staff at all, but if you send me females let 'em be steady, sensible ones, I said to the Nursing Officer. And what do I get? Young Mona Wynn who'd try and flirt with Johnny Glover and he's demented, and blind with it.'

Maybe Wynn looked flighty and maybe her uniform was too tight. Maybe she wore too much make-up and had a gleam in her eye. But she was sharp and efficient and had passed her nursing exams with distinctions, so what was he getting at?

'This. What I'm getting at is this, Doctor Delaney. There's too much familiarity between Nurse Wynn and Doctor Stafford. Giggling and whispering together. Having lunch together. Calling each other by christian names. It's not right, Doctor Delaney, and it's bad for ward discipline. It'll lead to trouble, with Doctor Stafford being married and trying to make a career for himself. I know he's only a locum and so he should be watching his step if he wants to get on in this hospital. It won't do him no good.'

What a prurient old woman Latimer was becoming. I was mad with him for his prudish moaning, especially coming after Manners. Why didn't he have a word with Wynn himself? Tell her to watch it while on duty?

'I did.' Latimer banged the desk so hard it shook. 'I had her in here and read the riot act to her and do you know what she said? Stood there as bold as brass and told me not to be so suburban.'

Latimer's jowls wobbled with rage. 'So I had a go at Doctor Stafford,' he went on. 'I put my arm around him and I talked to him man to man like he was my own son. He's that open and honest, Doctor Stafford, that he makes you feel protective. Seems to have no thought to what people think. I said to him, I said, it's up to you to make people respect you, and they do, everyone agrees that you're a good doctor, but consider, I said, consider how it'll look to others, if you go mooning over a young woman like Nurse Wynn. Talked to him for an hour I did. I never did speak to a medical officer like I spoke to him, but at the end of it all he just looked at me and smiled and do you know what he said?'

I shook my head.

'"Doctors are only human, Mr Latimer. And Nurse Wynn's a very pretty girl, as well as being a good nurse." That's what he said. He doesn't seem to have a care to his reputation, to what people will think and say. And you know what hospital gossip is like.'

The door burst open and a young male nurse with eyes popping like a surprised frog's said that a patient called Bill Martin had swallowed a pin.

'More like ten pints of beer in the Nag's Head.' Latimer snapped, and said he'd attend to the patient in a minute.

On the way out I told Latimer that I was sure there was nothing in Oliver's attention to Nurse Wynn, nothing more than he'd said, just appreciation of a pretty girl. I'd tell him to be more careful, I lied. I couldn't bring myself to mention gossip like that to Oliver. It really wasn't any of my business as nothing had happened, nothing more than two people registering attraction. But I couldn't discount Latimer's sense of danger. There was the time he had warned about a fire-raiser and nobody paid attention until after one ward had to be evacuated when a bed caught fire; the period when drugs went missing and Latimer put an unerring finger on the nurse who was a junkie; the occasion when one of our most intelligent, alcoholic patients was mysteriously getting drunker and drunker in spite of being specialled by a non-stop rota of nurses, and it was Latimer who'd copped that the glass of water containing the patient's false teeth was in fact vodka. No, Mr Latimer might be a boring fusspot at times but he wasn't to be discounted.

I was so wound up and worried after doing some shopping that I phoned Frankie later in the evening and told her about the gossip. 'I can't understand it,' I said. 'Unless there's something very wrong with the marriage, and they seem to be very fond of each other, Olwyn and Oliver.'

'Never can tell.' Frankie said sagely. 'Bed isn't everything, but it can be a hell of a lot in marriage. I mean, if it's not right, nothing else is. I sound very Irish but what I mean is that in spite of being lovey-dovey looking, the Staffords may have problems.'

'Problems?'

Surely not. I hadn't heard or seen any fighting. All seemed perfect peace in the Stafford ménage. Not that it was any of my concern, except that Stafford worked for me and if there was any funny business I didn't want it on my wards.

'I don't want to have to talk to him about it. You know, seen to be nosey and snoopy. I just don't want trouble,' I said.

'Then ignore it. Carry on as usual. It's a generation gap thing,' Frankie said. 'You and me missed out both ways. We were young in the buttoned-up inhibited era and now we could be swingers, we're into the Roaring Forties and fodder for euthanasia.'

'Speak for yourself.' I said. 'Of course patients are something else,' I added, and told her of my worry that Oliver was getting too involved with Coralie Kane and that was dynamite.

'He'd never be such a bloody fool,' Frankie said crisply. 'It's just that he likes women, and shows it.'

'Underneath the surface fripperies Coralie is steel,' I remarked.

'And Oliver's a good psychiatrist and realises it. You're getting a bit dotty about all this, Joyce. Have a good sleep, you're probably jiggered and not seeing straight. Till Saturday.'

Dotty. Not seeing straight. Frankie always dealt from the shoulder. I tried to recover some lost sleep but I kept straining to hear the Staffords. Come to think of it their bedroom was right under mine and I'd never heard anything, not a laugh or a voice. The walls of the old house weren't that thick. Maybe the Staffords didn't sleep together at all? After tossing and turning and efforts to persuade myself that all was well and I was worrying unduly, I finally fell asleep.

Chapter Eleven

I wasn't looking forward to the meal at Frankie's one little bit. With all my fears about Oliver and the mess he seemed to be getting into, deliberately inviting even, I was very angry with him. Angry that his emotional maturity didn't measure up more to his real and outstanding skill as a doctor. But I hadn't seen my old friends for a few days and there was the matter of Barney's mysterious and grumbling indigestion. It must be some bug he picked up in India, I told Oliver, as we drove to Frankie's. We really could have walked but the forecast was for more rain and Olwyn looked so glamorous I felt it would be a shame to mess up her dress. Her hair, black and cloudy, hung loose and what with clever eye make-up and skilful use of blusher and a very pale rose lipstick, she could be a model, I told her. Even Oliver had taken some trouble and he looked dashing in a blue suit and a red tie.

Barney seemed lively enough and pranced around doing what he loved, pouring out enormous drinks for everyone. Frankie appeared from the kitchen resplendent in her peacock kaftan. She said she hoped we liked garlic because she had put some in the goulash. Before Barney could say a word she swiftly added that she'd kept his separate goulash garlic free.

'Bloody good job,' said Barney seating himself beside Olwyn. He loved beautiful women and stared at her with such open admiration it had a sort of innocence. I could see that Olwyn was impressed with him. His quiff of white hair along with his handsome profile and booming voice made up to a real and devastating presence.

I hoped he wouldn't get too obvious in his appreciation of

Olwyn because after all these years and the tempestuous rows, Frankie could become uncharacteristically jealous. A trait she'd never ever showed with her other men.

'All this tummy trouble is due to the sand in my stomach. Got dysentery during the war, you see,' Barney added, fixing Olwyn with his bold blue eyes.

Frankie appeared again to tell us the meal was ready. And what a meal. Frankie had excelled herself and gave us a salmon mousse, followed by goulash so excellent that we all had a second helping, regretting it when a melting chocolate pudding arrived. Barney was in top form, spinning around charging everyone's glasses and he and Frankie were almost billing and cooing.

'Yes. I flatter myself I know far more about my innards then any doctor.' Barney was expansive. Helping himself to more port he unburdened himself about the medical profession. 'All right if they have to open a gut or take out a lump. They're crude barber surgeons really.'

As he got into his favourite subject I saw Frankie frown and I knew the jut of her chin meant trouble, especially when Barney took no notice of her calling. 'Shut up for God's sake, Barney. You're worse than any doctor for talking medical shop. Olwyn and Oliver are here to forget about hospitals and patients. They don't want to sit and listen to you going on about your indigestion.'

But Oliver let her down by saying that he was very interested in Barney's symptoms, so Frankie swooped on Olwyn and me with a glance, and said we'd have our brandy in comfort in the sitting-room. As she disappeared to make the coffee I thought great, here's a chance for me to talk to Olwyn on her own, but just as I was going to start putting out feelers Oliver appeared looking grave.

'Barney's not so well, Frankie. He's a bit dizzy and faint . . .'

Frankie could move with amazing speed for a big woman. 'Too much port,' she said. But suddenly she was grey and worried looking as she dashed out after Oliver.

'He looked so very well,' Olwyn said. 'Sort of blooming with health. The last person you'd imagine would want a doctor really. Of course, he's not young is he?'

No, I said, swirling my brandy around. No, Barney wasn't young and hadn't been well lately. Only he was a great hypochondriac and so one had to beware of a 'Wolf Wolf' syndrome.

'And they seem so happy together. Maybe it's because they aren't married.'

I hadn't time to wonder about this cynical and cryptic comment because Frankie rushed in with a distrait and desperate expression saying that Barney was very ill and Oliver and she were taking him to St Basil's.

While she phoned the hospital I dashed out to the dining-room where Oliver was kneeling beside Barney who was lying flaccidly on the floor with a cushion under him. His face was mauve-coloured and he breathed with a laboured and whistling intensity.

'Frankie was for keeping him here a while but I think I know what's the matter with him and he's going to need full investigation and treatment,' Oliver said.

'For what? A coronary? Or is this his chest trouble back again?'

Oliver was loosening Barney's tie very gently. How stringy the neck, and I could barely get a pulse at the wrist. He was dying, my old friend, I knew it. He'd never, ever make the journey, short as it was to St Basil's, I whispered to Oliver. If it weren't cardiac pulmonary, I said, what else could it be?

'He's been dosing himself for months with whopping great dollops of bicarb,' Oliver said. 'I think he's shot his blood chemistry to hell and is in fact suffering from acidosis.'

'Meaning that the balance of acids in his blood has escalated and has put him into a coma?'

'That's what I think.'

'But Oliver, if this is true can the condition be rectified? Is it reversible?'

'Yes, I think so. But it'll take time and he'll need careful laboratory checking and monitoring. I've told Frankie to get on to Doctor Carson who runs the Metabolic Unit at St Basil's. He has a particular interest in biochemistry and his unit is first class.'

I stood looking down on Barney who seemed to have physically crumpled, cheeks sucked in and chin jutting out like a moribund Jack Frost. I just couldn't see any resurrection for my old friend, especially after the ambulance came and the men gently transferred him to a stretcher. Eyes rolling and turning up, he looked like the sort of wandering octogenarian who gets knocked down after blind jay-walking. Funny, I always imagined Barney would go out roaring damnation and defiance at the barber surgeons, not like this, an inanimate heap of old bones.

Frankie appeared looking distracted, unable to be comforted by Oliver, who was telling her that he'd go with Barney and phone her immediately there was any news. She grabbed his sleeve, her make-up stood out on her white face like foolish crayon marks put there by a shaky hand. Barney wouldn't make it, there was hardly a pulse, she groaned.

As the ambulancemen arranged Barney's stretcher in the back and the engine began to rev up she said piteously, 'Suppose he goes . . . dies on the way. We've never been separated really. I should go . . .'

Her hair had come loose, tumbling over her bent shoulders. Oliver put an arm around her. Better if she stayed, he said and she was to try not to worry, he'd phone as soon as he could.

As the ambulance whisked away I asked Frankie to make more coffee. It would help her to have something to do. Willy didn't even try to follow her and I went back to Olwyn. I told her what Oliver thought might be the matter.

'He's a good diagnostician,' she remarked.

'A good doctor,' I added.

I found everything a bit unreal, out of a surrealistic semi-dream state. It had all happened with the speed of a street accident. One minute Barney had been sitting, rubicund and gay and the next minute he'd lapsed into a coma. But he hadn't been well. The cough and chest symptoms no more than a red herring. Oliver was well up in all the recent advances on which Frankie and myself were rusty, and I hadn't seen him make a clinical boob yet but I thought he was wrong. I didn't base this hunch on concrete clinical signs, it was more an inner hunch based on years of experience in which you learned, as a doctor, to think of the common things and outrule them, before going on to the more exotic abnormalities due to, what had Oliver said, 'Self-dosing resulting in disturbed blood acid basis?' Oh no. An old man, and Barney had looked withered and shrunken under the red blanket, an old man was a thousand times more likely to be suffering from one of the very common degenerative diseases such as arteriosclerosis and cardio-vascular disease.

Olwyn, sitting beside me, looked sympathetic but her swathes of shiny dark hair and lovely, almost alabaster skin, were in cruel contrast to my last memory of Barney and I couldn't bear it. Why the hell didn't Oliver phone? They must surely have reached the hospital by now. And where was Frankie with the coffee?

I got up and rushed out to the kitchen. There was Frankie hunched on a chair beside the big table that had a list no matter what was done to it. Barney had said he was going to get it cut up for firewood but like so many things in Garland House nobody had ever got round to doing anything about it. Frankie was cradling one of Barney's shirts. He was most particular about the ironing of these and after years of strife Frankie had learned to do them to his liking. Tears were dripping down her face making snakes in her make-up, and her mouth looked swollen and smudged with lipstick from licking the tears away. Her hair fell down her back in two heavy ropes and I saw, now that I was close to her, how much white there was in it. She stared at me unseeing.

'He was always going on about the Big Death Scene. Wondering how he'd go. Death was one of his hobbies . . .'

That was true. As Frankie said, Barney, as well as his feud with the medical profession, could be ghoulishly pre-occupied with mortality. He got a morbid kick, we used to think, about out-living contemporaries and yet was it so morbid? When we reached his age maybe survival, every day of it, would be a cause for celebration.

'I thought about his dying. I couldn't help it, living with him, but I never, ever really thought it would *happen* .'

Frankie leaned over the shirt as if she wanted to get close to something that Barney had worn, wanted to ingest what was left of him. So close they were, I wondered, as I'd done on many occasions, why they hadn't got married? Maybe that was part of Frankie's grief now, but her next words confounded me.

'I love him. I'd give him my heart's blood. He has asked me about marriage often. Quite often. But I've *had* paper contracts. But now, I think he's gone, Joyce. I don't think I'll ever get over it.'

I was stunned by Frankie's deep and lacerating grief. Was this the insouciant woman, the female buccaneer of the emotions who had often had me in stitches with her cynical comments on life and men, especially men. How many times had she not chuckled over Shaw's dictum that love is the delusion that one man or woman is different to another? Yet here she was, crying into Barney's old shirt and calling her grief. Barney hadn't died. Maybe it was as Oliver said and then something could be done, I said.

'Listen . . .' she rolled tear-stained, almost black eyes at me. There was a touch of the old cynicism of Frankie as she blew her nose and put the shirt away. 'You and me, Joyce know well that Barney's had it. You . . .'

She was interrupted by Olwyn whose face had a most uncharacteristic flush of excitement. Oliver had phoned to say they'd arrived, Barney was being examined by the houseman and Carson was on his way in. Oliver would phone again when there was a new development. That meant, I thought frantically, that if Oliver didn't phone the news was bad. Then I decided that that was sloppy thinking due to worry and strain and that we could all do with coffee. Olwyn and I made the coffee and Frankie poured some more brandy for us, saying she herself wanted to keep her head clear but I persuaded her to take some and was glad I did so because time passed and there was no call from Oliver. We sat, the caffeine in the coffee had woken us, and we were alert but too tense for conversation. So strained that we tried to avoid looking at each other. There was nothing to say, I thought, no comforting clichés that wouldn't be an insult to Frankie's sorrow.

Once or twice she said things like: 'As long as he's not left paralysed or incontinent,' and I had an instant, horrific vision of a dribbling, vegetable with tubes sticking out of every orifice. Oh yes, there were worse things than death, Frankie and I both knew that, and so we sat glassy-eyed and tried not to think of the patients we'd seen and the things that were done to them in the name of medicine and research. There was even the new horror of organ transplant making resuscitation sometimes suspect. But poor Barney's organs, especially his kidneys, were too well-used to be of any help as re-treads.

'More coffee?' Olwyn asked us. Even after tonight with its traumas and keeping this vigil (it was now three o'clock) she looked coolly fresh. But she was young like Sheena and had the same reserves of stamina.

Frankie had just blearily asked what time it was, when the phone rang and she leaped up and fled to the sitting-room. Olwyn and I sat at attention, silent in our fear. But when Frankie rushed in she looked electric. Carson had been, had examined Barney, and agreed with Oliver. There had to be lots of tests and investigations but Carson had given his opinion that after some days of treatment Barney would be all right, though he was still unconscious now.

'The old devil's done it himself with all that bloody medicine he got from the chemist. Wouldn't see anyone after the mix up with the X-rays. Thank God!' Frankie said.

We sat, the three of us, bruised and bashed by the night's events, but now, as dawn was breaking, feeling that we had emerged from the nightmare and had made it into a new promise of life and hope. I don't remember what we said or indeed if we said anything at all but I remember, when at last we saw Frankie dozing, that Olwyn and I crept away.

Oliver hadn't returned from the hospital and Olwyn asked me in for some more coffee. I didn't want it. I didn't want anything but a bath and bed but this was the only opportunity to talk to Olwyn of my fears about his behaviour. And to have to do it now, after Oliver had been so marvellous with Barney, was cruel luck. On the other hand, the exhibition of his clinical skill could be said to pave the way for an expression of what was troubling me. So I sat, sipping coffee as the big old kitchen filled with the cold fingers of dawn. 'Oliver was a brick tonight, Olwyn. Absolutely marvellous.'

'It's what he's good at. So soaked in medicine that there's no question of it being just a job with him. It's his life. Simple as that.'

Or as complicated, I thought as Olwyn began to stroke Satan the cat. I told her, as I had told her before, that I valued and appreciated Oliver's work and wanted him to stay on, wanted them both to stay on.

She jumped up, scattering the cat and began to walk up and down, frenetic in her pacing. 'And don't you think that's what I want? It's what we need, Oliver and me. Some peace.'

Here it was, the hinting of secret fires and hurts. It didn't need a psychiatrist to gauge that all wasn't well with the Staffords.

'Oliver's being a bit indiscreet, Olwyn.' I began. Then I came right out with it, explaining that he seemed to be spending too much time with a very dangerous patient called Coralie Kane. Yes, the woman who had phoned. I wasn't implying that Oliver was doing anything wrong, he just wasn't allowing for the malice of Coralie who spelled trouble, and trouble was what Oliver could do without, especially if he wanted to apply for a job in Barrington or to stay on in his present position. Maybe I should have warned Oliver more positively, but privately I felt I'd done more than enough in that direction.

After that it was odd that she didn't look more stunned, I thought; bad enough to hear about your husband's dalliance without the added danger of a serious breach of the doctor-patient relationship.

She stood looking at me for a moment and then went out. She came back a few moments later with a sheaf of letters. No need for her to tell me that they were from Coralie, I knew that wavery writing in purple ink. I skimmed through them after Olwyn handed them to me; Coralie certainly had gone to town with these. They were typical of her theatricality: 'Always pestering me for sex'; 'Just like every other man'; 'the one thing on his mind'; and Oliver was named on every page.

'How long have you had these, Olwyn?'

'Over the past few weeks.'

'Does Oliver know of them?'

'No.'

He would have to know, and as soon as possible. Well, my worst fears were realised. In some queer way I was glad the waiting was over and that things were coming to a head. At the same time though, I was full of sick dread. I didn't dare think whether what Mrs Kane wrote was true, that Oliver had pestered her for sex. Most of the letters were just wild diatribes about men with no concrete accusations; but they could come later. This woman must be stopped, I told Olwyn, must be dealt with or she'd damage what after all was a doctor's work permit, his reputation.

'I'll make some coffee,' Olwyn sighed.

Heavily and automatically she went about her task. She was like a robot, I thought, unless she's just too shocked to react. But damn it, she's had these letters some time. Surely she must know the danger of a woman who was prepared to act out her fantasies in writing. At least, I assumed they were fantasies; to imagine anything else was beyond me at the moment.

'You are wondering why I'm so calm?' Olwyn asked as she set down coffee before me. 'It's not that I'm not the jealous kind. It . . . jealousy eats at me at times. I'm like a cat, a spitting cat with very sharp talons. It's just that I'm . . . I feel I have no call to indulge those feelings now. I told you before that I'm at fault, responsible for Oliver's unhappiness.'

What was she on about? This was no time for maudlin sentimental nonsense. She wasn't tight and didn't seem to be angry, but I wasn't in the mood for marriage guidance or counselling. There was Coralie to be dealt with, and soon, yet here was this girl mooning on about her marriage. I was tired, cross and impatient. But Olwyn seemed to be taken up, transfixed almost, with her thoughts. She moved to the window where dawn was splashing the sky with yellow and orange streaks.

'I'll have to tell you something to show you why I feel that this is all my fault, this Kane business. Oh, Oliver has an eye for women. I find him attractive so I realise that other women will, too. Do you remember talking about Haxton when you asked about references? From what I said you'll probably have guessed that I had an affair there.'

'Yes. Yes, it did occur to me,' I said.

'And it was an affair, short and transient and very unsatisfactory.'

Nothing new in that, for God's sake, I fumed to myself. I'd heard it all before. How the husband spent more and more time at work neglecting the wife whose days became more lonely and sad. Then the meeting with a new man who had affection and attention to pour on the wife's parched love life. The glorious, passion filled days, the guilty agony. I knew it all and wanted to shout at Olwyn, who surely wasn't naïve enough to think I hadn't come across this hoary chestnut. Instead of indulging her guilt and shame, giving in to some inner compulsion to spill beans which would be better left in the bag, she should be getting down to basics and helping me to deal with bloody Coralie.

'Oliver found out, of course.' She said dully.

I nearly said, but don't they usually? I was bored and fed up with this whole subject. I got enough seedy revelations from patients and I certainly didn't want to have to work with a man whose wife didn't just have a small fling but insisted on talking about it, too.

'But of course it was *who* I slept with that would really have hurt Oliver.' She went on. She gave me a long, almost calculating look as if she was actually daring me to draw conclusions.

Well, here it comes, I thought, now for the revelation about whoever it was had taken her fancy. But her next words riveted me. I couldn't have been more surprised if she had whipped out a gun from her stocking top, Bond style.

'It was Coulter. Felix Coulter.' She said flatly.

I had a bizarre and repellent vision of Felix in the throes of orgiastic passion and I must have looked as if I'd been struck with a wet kipper. Olwyn continued, in that level, sing-song Welsh voice, that of course she knew I'd be surprised, she'd been amazed herself.

'Just one of those things, like the song. And too hot not to cool down. Felix came over to Haxton from time to time you see, and he was very unsettled in his job here, trying to finalise going to America and I didn't think things were too happy at home. How do these things happen? I can only say that Felix and I met when we were both unsettled, at a loose end as it were.'

Possible, but still hard to imagine, my thoughts ran. But wasn't much of one's friends' sex lives funny and unlikely? And it still didn't explain why Coulter had helped to get Oliver Stafford to work here in Barrington. Why hadn't they stayed at Haxton, I asked?

'I wanted out because I felt there was less chance of Oliver getting to hear about Felix over here,' Olwyn said. 'You see, it wasn't love between Felix and me, it was the sort of intense thing which sometimes happens on holiday and at parties. No question of permanency or anything, I know that doesn't excuse me, makes it worse really, but both Felix and I felt very guilty even after it was all over, and I think Felix wanted to do a good turn to Oliver.'

'How come?'

'Well. Oliver was working latterly in Haxton with a young consultant who was very hard to get on with. He lorded it over Oliver. Everyone said so. And I know how unhappy Oliver was. Couldn't get it out of him for ages. Maybe that's why I drifted into that thing with Coulter, because Oliver was so depressed. I don't know. But I felt we ought to move over here. And Oliver is happy here, Joyce, and he likes working with you. Now you know about me you probably think I'm a little tramp. But I love Oliver and I feel I've let him down, so how can I possibly be angry about Coralie Kane?'

I made myself as brisk and no nonsense as possible and told her to shut up about what she'd done in the past. Coulter was gone and I wouldn't tell anyone, not even Frankie. Neither must she. What we had to do was to try and work something out to beat Coralie. Olwyn managed to draw strength from somewhere and pull herself back to reality. When should we speak to Oliver, she asked. Just as soon as possible, I said. I'd wait till he came back from St Basil's.

Olwyn heated up the coffee which had gone cold and after she'd given me a cup she hugged me and said, 'I'm very sorry you've been dragged into this, Joyce. You've been very kind to us both and I'm sorry we've brought you nothing but trouble.' That wasn't true I said. After all, Oliver had found Melinda and had managed Barney so well last night. It was too late for tears or blame. Too late for anything except to hope that Coralie had got what she wanted; to deliver a swipe to another of the hated male sex. We could only hope that the spiteful letters and the expressed malice were all Coralie was going to stir up because, if she took things further, plenty of fat would be used to make the fire a holocaust. Oliver must be warned forthwith, I said. Not only must he never see Mrs Kane again but he must get in touch with his Defence Society right away. Their function, for which each doctor paid a hefty anuual subscription, was to deal with accusations of negligence, malpractice and cases of unprofessional associations. All complaints, in short, which could lead to erasure from the register.

'You don't think there's a danger of that?' Olwyn was sickly pale, almost gaunt. She shook back her fall of hair and smoothed a few strands from her face with hands which were now shaking.

Just then Oliver came in, tired but buoyant. 'Barney's still in coma, but not so deeply. He's got all sorts of drips up and is in the Intensive Care but expected to come out of it later today. Of course he's to have all manner of weird and wonderful tests, but he'll survive. Carson is terribly interested and thanked me . . .' Oliver sat down and Olwyn turned away, bending over the coffee percolator. Oliver stiffened, his glance flying from me to his wife. 'Come on, what's the matter? We should all be crazy mad with joy about Barney . . . that he's surviving . . .'

As his voice trailed away I said, 'Yes. I'm afraid there is more trouble, Oliver. Coralie Kane's been writing to Olwyn . . .'

As Olwyn put down a coffee cup in front of him he grabbed her. 'What's this Ol? You're not taking some daft letters from a patient to heart are you? There's mad you are yourself . . .'

There was a sharp exchange in Welsh between the two of them. I got the word 'tup' which I knew meant 'mad' in Welsh. They were rattled. Olwyn looked more sad than worried but Oliver, for almost the first time since I'd known the man, seemed very angry. I gathered that he thought Olwyn was over-reacting from the way he was talking crossly to her as he read the letters she'd bashfully given him and then flung them down again.

'She's that worst of women, Ol. Her aggression is her defence. And she's paranoid, too.'

'Then you should be careful with her, not spend too much time with with her.'

There, Olwyn had said it for me. Now more than Stafford's asperity I was surprised by her waspish tone. But why should I be? The ramifications and permutations of relationships were paraded in front of me every day by my patients. One thing I was sure of now, Olwyn was not just a complacent wife. I had to be sure of something else though.

'This I must know, Oliver,' I said. 'Is there any substance, anything more than paranoia in what Mrs Kane is on about?'

Olwyn was gathering up the letters distastefully as if they contained some fungoid growth and Oliver looked at me through eyes that could sometimes appear hazel, sometimes, like now, almost brown. He looked shaken but his gaze was direct. Nothing, nothing in what Mrs Kane said other than the ploys of a sex starved woman who, because of her hysterical personality demanded attention at all times and at all costs.

'So. Nothing in what she said?' I asked, and he shook his head.

I was wishing Olwyn didn't look so worried, when Oliver said he wanted to ask me about the registrar's job. He was thinking of applying and hoped he could use me as a referee. The job hadn't been advertised yet, I said, but he had to remember that eyes were watching him. The fact that Coralie had revealed her malice in writing to his wife should show him what she was capable of. And he wasn't to see her again, I would take over. His reference from me would depend on his behaviour for the next few weeks. I felt school marmish, fussy old square, but more than ever, now that Olwyn had shown me the pattern of Oliver's behaviour, I knew that he was skating on almost melting ice and seemed to lack all protective survival tactics. Even now, after what I'd said and what he must have suspected Olwyn told me, he sat back over his coffee and regaled us with Barney's condition, how it started, showed itself and how it was to be treated. Watching him, full of vigour and enthusiasm for clinical niceties I felt a surge of rage that his personal conduct and dangerously irresponsible behaviour were so at odds with his medical acumen. I had warned him. Mr Latimer had warned him, and he knew now he was in potential trouble with Coralie Kane, yet I had a horrible feeling that either what I'd said hadn't gone home or else would be disregarded. And from Olwyn's sad, resigned expression as she showed me out I knew that she felt that, too.

Chapter Twelve

It wasn't worth going to bed. I went back to my own flat feeling as if I'd been beaten with sticks. My talk with the Staffords had increased my gloomy presentiment of danger rather than lessened it. Olwyn was emerging as the sharper, more realistic and probably stronger partner. She realised how tenuous Oliver's position was in the hospital, how damaging any scandal would be to him now that he was interested in applying for a permanent job. But she was to some extend blinded into inaction by her deep and scarring shame at her inability to be what she'd called 'a real woman' and a 'proper wife' to her husband. So immature was Oliver's behaviour, so out of place with his skills as a doctor, that I was beginning to wonder how much of a 'real man' Oliver was and thinking that it was time she, Olwyn, stopped feeling guilty and blaming herself.

Still, as I sat drinking tea, I thought about the events of the night. Commitment to patients could be tiring and trying but dealing with the emotions of one's friends and colleagues was totally exhausting. I'm on duty all the bloody time, I couldn't help feeling, and the repository for everyone's griefs and pains. I must have been very exhausted and nearly forgot that I'd promised to phone Sheena.

When I heard her say how marvellous she felt, how grateful she was for everything, I felt mean and sour especially when she told me to be sure to tell her about Wendy. I then rang the police who said that Wendy had been seen, had given a statement and that's as much as they knew. No action had been taken yet anyway. And they'd sent a policewoman around to get the statement, Constable Wiggin told me.

Now for Frankie. She was back from a dash to the hospital where she'd been allowed a brief look at Barney.

'He looks all shrunken, lying there so quietly. It's just not him to allow all those needles and tubes to be stuck into him. You know how he'd create if he was . . .' She stopped.

I knew she'd been going to say 'alive' so I reminded her that wasn't the main thing, and the thing to be thankful for was that the acidosis was treatable.

'I know,' she said humbly. 'It's just that it's all happened so suddenly. He was sparkling, full of life and then next thing he was gone . . .'

The doctor in Frankie had vanished and she was all woman, and a loving woman, at the moment, Not that her feminine instincts were buried too far; it was just that, like me, she'd found it left you too exposed not to have some sort of hide, some sort of defence against the sick and the suffering. If you got involved, let your withers be wrung too often, you cracked and sometimes broke.

'I'll never be able to thank Oliver,' Frankie said. 'He's . . . well . . . he's a very, very good doctor. You're lucky to have him working for you.'

'Yes,' I said.

I mustn't have sounded too sure because Frankie asked what was the matter and I said I was just a bit tired and could she call to see me on her way home from the hospital tonight? If she wasn't too jaded herself. I would have some steak and onions, I said, because I knew she was particularly partial to steak. She'd be delighted, she said, but she wouldn't stay late. I told her to give Barney a kiss from me and I'd be down to see him just as soon as he was allowed visitors. I got a shock when I realised that it was nearly eleven o'clock. Time was doing the funny things it does when people get caught up in unusual events, so I threw on my clothes and set off for the hospital.

When I got to Gilbert Ward Mr Latimer drew me into an office that was rarely used and said with an air of mystery that he'd spoken to Nurse Wynn. Given her, as he said, 'an 'eavy dressing down', made a last appeal to her on the grounds that Stafford wanted to get a job in the hospital and temptation mustn't be put in his way. He'd been expecting a toss of the head and a 'Mind your own business' rebuff, but to his surprise Nurse Wynn had taken it quite well. Probably because one of the senior nursing staff had now come to hear of the association and Wynn was shrewdly aware of this. After all, it was not as if Oliver and Wynn were young and foolish, Latimer rumbled in his most magisterial tones.

Next, there was Coralie to be tackled. Down at St Basil's I asked Morgan to find out for me when Coralie Kane had her next appointment with Doctor Stafford. She could tell me that without the book, Morgan said. Mrs Kane was seen every week by Doctor Stafford, but she had a late appointment, at six o'clock when the other patients had gone. I must have looked a bit shaken because Morgan, who had an acute sense for vocal nuance, asked me sharply whether there was anything the matter?

'No. Not yet,' I said. The niggling worry about Oliver was growing into a continuous gnawing fear that obtruded into my every thought; even when I met Oliver next day and he looked almost cheery telling me about an interesting case of an asthmatic who'd gone psychotic on steroids. He was either a compulsive liar or didn't appreciate his professional fragility. What good was it being a smart diagnostician, I thought, as Oliver told me about how well Barney was doing, if he had such a kamikaze attitude to his professional reputation? He reeled off all the drugs Barney was on and told me about meeting and accompanying Carson on his rounds. Doctor Carson, he said, had just attended a conference in Amsterdam on disturbances in blood chemistry, where there had been much discussion on the self-induced states of acidosis. Oliver quoted article after article, study after study.

'I'm going to phone the library in the British Medical

Association. I often use them . . .' He was just about to disappear, and, of anyone I'd known, Oliver could vanish in a split second. It was as if he had his own private trap door. But I was determined to underline what I'd said about Coralie Kane. He wasn't to see her again. I'd take over and that was an order.

'Sure. Sure,' he said vaguely and dashed out.

Well. I'd done all I could. There wasn't anything more to do that I could think of. One quarter of what I'd said to Oliver would have shattered a normal doctor. Maybe Oliver was too used to tight corners. Well, I hoped he was good at getting out of them. For himself and for Olwyn's sake.

I didn't get home till almost seven and I was in the middle of beating the T-bones when Frankie arrived bearing a bottle of champagne.

'I just thought to hell with it, we need something to cheer us up. Shall I open it?'

I said yes, and added that I gathered Barney was on the up?

'Up is the word,' she said as the cork gave the ritual 'pop'. 'Conscious, out of the ICU and giving hell to the nurses. Even cursing . . .'

She passed me a glass of champagne and I said he had to be all right if the swearing had returned.

'That's it. "What the hell?" going on all the time. Thinks of course that he only had a "weakness" as he calls it and that everyone's making too much fuss. I didn't bother to argue. I just hope that Carson will sort him out about poisoning himself again. I had a look around his room this morning and there's bloody great boxes of empty powders and mixtures. He must have spent a fortune at the chemist. And the cunning hawk didn't go to just one chemist but spread his trade. I threw them all out.'

I put the steaks to grill and began to toss lettuce with French dressing. Probably because I'd not had lunch and little sleep, the glass of champagne was making me feel woozy but it was a lovely wooziness and Frankie refilled my glass.

'I shall never, ever be able to thank Oliver enough. Maybe the illness would have been diagnosed eventually. But maybe not. It could have been too late. It's funny, you don't realise what things mean to you till they're nearly taken away. And I'm so fond of Barney. I'll never fight with him again. I mean it. Never.'

'Go on. You both enjoy it. The fire's there when the sparks fly. You're both fiery people, Frankie.'

'Maybe so. Oh . . . I left some champers with Olwyn. Just as a token. I thought she looked ill. Any trouble?'

I said I'd tell her later. The steaks were done, sizzling and burnt outside and blue-red within, the way she liked them. We sat and ate in the kitchen, not speaking because we were both ravenous. I was glad because I didn't really want to tell her about Oliver. Somehow I didn't want to spoil a happy time like this when, full of good wine and tender beef, we could let out our mental stays, forgetting we were two middle-aged women who happened to be doctors, and surrender to a joy which was the more appreciated because it was rare.

'You know,' said Frankie, slicing some Brie, 'you know it doesn't do us any harm in some ways to experience again what it's like to have to depend on hospitals. To have a try and find out news, wait and worry and generally see things from the other end of the stethoscope. Makes you understand how patients and relatives feel. How they worry, imagine the worst and try to read gestures, expressions and tones of voice. When the Sister told me tonight that Barney was going to be all right I could have kissed her. On the way home I wanted to sing and shout. But I settled for buying champagne.'

I was hoping that in her exultation she'd forget to enquire about trouble. I'd even thought of fobbing her off, but I should have known better. She'd always been able to pump me, had been mistress of translating my expressions and when I was pouring the coffee she looked at me sharply and said, 'Spit it out. There's something up. I know it. It couldn't be about Barney. Melinda is restored to Sheena, so what is it? Has Wendy been on to you? Or that Pillsworth virago?'

Nobody. Skip it, I said.

But Frankie as she always did beat down my defences. 'You went home with Olwyn, Something happened. Come on. Out with it.'

So I told her and for a moment she was silent, shocked into dumbness by the sheer craziness of Oliver in allowing himself to be compromised by a patient like Coralie.

'I did warn him,' I said. 'Told him to watch it. But I'm sure there's nothing in it, Frankie. No more than his being too nice, too kind to Coralie not realising what a bitch she is.'

She couldn't fathom it, Frankie said, lighting a cigarette which she did only when very disturbed. She listened, nodding and blinking against the smoke when I told her about Olwyn's revelation. A strong lady, Frankie said, but still and all, not a cause for Oliver taking up with trouble in the form of Coralie. Especially when he obviously was attractive to women like Mona Wynn.

'I rather like Wynn,' Frankie said. 'She was a junior nurse when I worked at Barrington but she was damn good in spite of her sex-pot appearance. And not malicious. I wouldn't mind what that old puritan Latimer says about her. Just because she's sultry looking with bedroom eyes doesn't mean she isn't good at her job.' Of course, Frankie went on, morals being so few and fluid today who the hell cared? But messing with patients was suicidal for a doctor. That still held. Especially if, like Oliver, you were hoping to get a permanent job.

'But is he?' she demanded. 'Is Oliver really wanting to

settle and put down roots or is this a sop to Olwyn who wants just that? Maybe she was getting broody and wanted a family.'

I was simply bursting to shake Frankie by telling her about Olwyn's affair with Coulter but I held back, basely and superstitiously fearing that I'd get a lashing from the fates if I broke my word to Olwyn.

'People never tell you the whole truth,' Frankie said more pointedly than she realised. 'I bet that sly boots Coulter knew a great deal. Something happened at Haxton and Stafford had to be got off someone's back.'

Sure, I said, but the main thing now was to get Coralie Kane to lay off because Stafford would disappear down a very big hole if she didn't. I told Frankie that I'd warned Oliver, hoping I'd put the fear of God into him, and that I was going to see Mrs Kane myself and inform her that she wasn't to see Doctor Stafford again.

'Oh God, Frankie,' I said. 'I'm choked with trouble and drama. There's been nothing else since the Staffords came.'

'Could be coincidental,' Frankie said, grabbing her bag. 'I'm off to phone Basil's to see how Barney's getting on. You've done all you can for Oliver. There's nothing more you can do except wait and see.'

That was what was so hard I said.

'Remember old Baldy O'Grady?' Frankie twisted her face into a semblance of the dusty professor. 'Till the cervix is fully dilated, masterly inactivity gentlemen, masterly inactivity.'

'I'm responsible, Frankie,' I said. 'As I'm legally in charge of the patients, and even though I passed Coralie to Oliver, I just have this feeling that things aren't going to end here. What if Coralie reports to the GMC?'

'She isn't bright enough to have heard of them and anyway what would she say? Look, Joyce, all that's happened is that Oliver has got over-involved with a patient. To listen to you anyone would imagine he'd slept with bloody Coralie. Belt up for God's sake. Just wait and see, there's nothing else you can do. See ya.'

Maybe my old friend was right. When we were students Frankie often called me Cassie because she said I was a true Cassandra, always shouting doom and gloom. Too like my father, she used to say, prone to seeing intimations of death and disaster everywhere. What I needed was a half day, I decided. I'd take one after disposing of Coralie.

I slept deeply and awoke more refreshed than I'd done for days. Sheena phoned to say she and Melinda were fit and well and when I phoned about Barney the nurse told me he was making excellent progress though still very weak. Something about the nurse's voice was familiar.

'Yes. It's Mona Wynn speaking,' she said. No mistaking the crack in the voice which was oddly attractive. 'I've been seconded to St Basil's to do my general training.'

Well, well, well, I thought, the PNO at Barrington had used the well-worn ploy of when there's trouble transfer the personnel involved. There was always a traffic in nurses between the hospitals of course but Nurse Wynn's transfer seemed a bit too coincidental to be innocent. Interesting to see how Barney got on with her. Well, I would say, unless Barney's penchant for badinage with a well-formed female was influenced by his illness.

My sleep, the bright day with its fresh breeze that made the sun's scorch less trying, and the prospect of my half day to be spent, I'd decided, in just moseying around the shops, pepped me up so much that I didn't even mind the usual glare in the clinic room. Nor the fact that Morgan had forgotten the table fan again. When she'd fetched it and apologised for not remembering because of two emergencies at midday I asked her whether Mrs Kane had arrived. No, said Morgan, but maybe Coralie knew already that Doctor Stafford wasn't going to see her? I said I didn't see how that could happen but then you never knew what patients had picked up, it was amazing how the gossip flew.

Just then Oliver appeared and after Morgan had bustled out I asked him about Coralie. Had he heard from her? Why hadn't she turned up today?

He smiled vaguely, eyes slithering away from me and I knew, knew deep down that he was lying. 'She doesn't always turn up,' he said. 'Gets one of her "turns" and decides to keep to the house.'

Not when she has a chance to see a doctor, especially a male one. But I didn't voice my thought.

'Or maybe she's feeling better. You know how unpredictable she is.'

All right, I said, but he was to remember. No more interviews with Mrs Kane. If she did surface I would deal with her. And discharge her. This time for good.

'Yes. O.K.' Oliver began to fiddle with a pen. He looked as if he wanted to say something. He's probably scared about whether I'm going to act as his referee, I thought, or maybe he's going to mention Mona Wynn. But he just asked me a few questions about Sheena and then moved on to Barney, how well he was getting on. Even able to take fluids by mouth soon. Had I seen him?

'No,' I said, 'I'll pop in on my way home from the clinic. It was very quick of you to spot that Barney was suffering from acidosis rather than a coronary.'

'Oh . . . I'd been reading up some stuff in the *New England Journal of Medicine*.'

I couldn't help asking him why, with his interest in medicine and his obvious knowledge, why he hadn't done his Membership?

'Just never got around to it,' he said, putting his pen away. 'I'm not much of a one for exams. Or anything competitive. I must lack the killer instinct!'

Maybe, I said, but he should remember that other people did have a killer instinct, people like Coralie Kane. His eyes flickered and looked away. Then he got up and said he had a patient waiting.

I was quite glad in a way that Coralie failed to turn up. I wasn't looking forward to seeing her. I'd always found her pretty infuriating, the more so now when I knew she'd been badgering Olwyn. It was typical of the Kane lack of thought for other people and their needs. Oh well, I would have to take Frankie's advice and stop worrying. I needed a rest, even if it was only a half day. Several of the patients enquired whether I was ill and when I did manage to peep in the mirror I could see what they meant. My face was creased with fatigue and my eyes dull. I put on some paint for Barney's sake and went out and bought some fruit for him remembering too late that fruit was too acid to be given to him.

The private wing at St Basil's was tucked behind the main part of the hospital. It was the source of continual rumour and speculation. It was going to be closed; the ancillary staff were going to boycott the building; the local MP, lobbied beyond endurance about élitism and privileges, was going to demand that the block be turned over to the local authorities for use as a community centre. Controversy burned and two consultants, depending on their private fees for educating their children in what they deemed the proper way, threatened to take up the offer of Saudi gold and were stopped only when the MP developed strangulated piles and was looked after so very well in the private wing that there was no more about its closure. Not that the patients in the private wing got any better treatment, but they did get a room of their own and unlimited visiting.

I checked in at Sister's office to find Mona Wynn sitting there. Her hair was a tangle of silver and ash curls by which her tiny starched cap was almost obscured, and she batted those incredible yellowy eyes at me.

'I've come to see Mr Osborne, that's if he's allowed to have visitors,' I said.

'Oh yes. Especially if the visitor is a doctor,' she said demurely and I handed her the fruit saying that it wasn't the best present for a patient suffering from hyperacidity. But I was sure she could use it.

'Thanks very much. I adore fruit,' she smiled. 'I agree it wouldn't be good for Mr Osborne. Doctor Carson has put him on a very rigid fluid intake while his metabolism gets back to normal. In fact, we were going to put him into the Metabolic Unit but it's full and no prospect of a bed. He's still having to be fed intravenously but we're hoping to start oral feeding tomorrow, and then it should be plain sailing until the body chemistry returns to normal.'

The goo-goo eyes and the mop of curls were an open invitation to a proposition at least. The wiggle of the hips under the flattering pink and white uniform could have made *Playboy*, but Wynn knew her medical onions all right. On the way down the passage to room ten, Barney's room, I asked how she liked a general hospital after a psychiatric one?

Oh, she said, tossing her curls, the standard of nursing was infinitely better at Barrington where patients were treated like human beings and not patronised and bullied as they were here at St Basil's. Psychiatric nurses studied their patients' personalities, took time off to talk to them and get to know them, but here it was all you could do to get through the unending bed-making, dressing, enemas and bedpans.

Probably not enough staff, or not enough money to pay them from the bankrupt NHS. Anyway, I thought, but didn't say, that she hadn't been at St Basil's long enough to judge, even though she was voicing what every other nurse we'd sent from Barrington had to say.

'Visitor for you Mr O.,' Wynn said.

Barney, who had been lying looking out of the window which showed nothing more than Yorkely's railway station, turned towards me. He had aged and looked shrunken. His cheeks hung flaccidly in definite dew laps and his eyes had lost their glitter. The thin tube running from his mouth was secured with plaster, making his speech difficult. When he moved he was impeded by the splints on his arm, which held the end of the tube attached to the up-ended drip bottle which allowed the saline and glucose mixture to drip slowly into the vein in his arm.

'Watch out . . . you'll have the fluid going into the tissues.' Wynn rushed forward and bent over his arm, her skirt up to expose a considerable view of black satin petticoat.

'Drip be buggered,' Barney said weakly and winked at me. 'I can tell you when I get my strength back I'm going to add a drop of whisky to that bottle.'

'Now. Now.' Wynn flashed him one of her most melting smiles. 'Didn't you do enough harm to yourself swallowing all those stomach powders? Doctor Carson says you're not to have any alcohol for weeks. Bad for the liver.'

'My liver's hob-nailed. Too pickled to be harmed,' Barney boomed as Wynn swished out. 'Great girl,' he added, as I sat down at the end of his bed. The room was small and functional and the view from the window most uninspiring. 'It's bloody lying here like a swaddled child. And I don't think much of the nurses. Now that girl who's gone out is grand. Never hurts you and has a way with her. Always glad when she's on. And there's a young West Indian, Nurse Pearl, who's a topper, too. But the rest of 'em, I wouldn't let them look after fowl.'

A big shake of salt to be taken, I knew. I could imagine how hellish Barney was to nurses and so his praise of Wynn was praise indeed. She'd told him a bit about herself. She was divorced and had to bring up two children on her own. As well as looking after her mother who had cancer and a father who was an alcoholic. She was far more than a pretty face.

'And that's something,' Barney grumbled. 'The others, except for Pearl, are a po-faced bunch. Oh, and there's a woman who cleans the room who's human. As for the doctors, well, Carson's all right. Doesn't say a word of course, just comes in and stares at me, and as for his houseman . . . well, he's a young Indian who seems to know no English. I told him I felt champion and he goggled at me and asked "Champion of what?" Jesus Christ . . .' Barney groaned and launched into a diatribe against hospitals and doctors.

He was getting no sleep, no rest, he grumbled, was woken at cock crow by clumsy young girls who stuck thermometers up his arm and did unspeakable things to his lower parts. He was about to ask me to throw the clothes back so he could show me his bottle and catheter but I was quick enough to say I knew what he meant. He'd just be recovering from the first assault on his person, he went on, when another batch of amazons descended and grabbed at him to take his pulse and blood pressure. If he tried to doze or rest he was interrupted by the clatter of the cleaning woman, and as soon as she went out he was trundled about by other clumsy nurses who made his bed and gave him a bed bath.

'It's all bloody go,' he ranted. 'Paper boys, porters, bloody women selling stamps and sweets. Sister, the doctor doing rounds, women crashing in to take your flowers back. I can't get five minute's peace in this bloody place. Of course it's better than the ICU. Mercifully, I was without my faculties when they put me there but when I woke up and found that I was wired up to an array of machines which looked like things from outer space and tubes stuck into every orifice, I gave them hell till they took me out. Christ, but hospitals have got worse since my day. Bloody worse. I suppose the only way poor bastards who are patients put up with it is that they're in no position to do otherwise. But I intend to take things further, write to the bloody minister if necessary. Christ, if they bring in euthanasia we can pack up. All this organ snatching is bad enough. I tell you, Joyce, down in that ICU it dawned on me that they didn't want me to get better really, but were just cossetting me to keep my kidneys going and give them to someone else. Oh, I know what they're up to, but no bugger's going to take my kidneys without a fight, I can tell you. I know their game . . .'

Barney was better. The Osborne spirit was back trumpeting away. To distract him, I said he mustn't generalise too much, look how Oliver had spotted what was the matter. No easy thing either, I said, because nobody had known how much indigestion mixture and tablets he'd been swallowing. Anyway, whatever he'd taken had altered the delicate balance of his blood chemistry which was now being rectified by the fluids going into his vein.

Yes, yes, he said testily, Frankie had explained all that to him, and given him hell for being dotty enough to stuff himself with remedies he'd bought at the chemist.

'Yes,' I said absently, 'and doctors are worst of all for self-medication. We have a saying; "He who is his own doctor is a fool."'

'Like solicitors making a hash of it when they try and make their own wills. Come on now, what's the news? I heard I heard all about Sheena, that happened before I got ill. Of course, I get the odd bit from Mona, but like Frankie, I don't think she wants to get me going. I'm fed up with being treated like a moronic child. It's so bloody boring lying here with a tube stuck up my arm and in my privates . . .'

I let him chunter on, it was better than having to stall his plea for gossip, whatever Frankie had told him, and I didn't think she'd said anything, I didn't want to discuss Oliver, even the talk about Mona. Now that I was seeing a bit more of her and was more clued in about her, I somehow felt she'd be loyal to Oliver, after it had been explained to her about his hopes for a permanent job. I was sure of one thing though, Mona's career came first with her, it had to if she had all those home troubles that Barney spoke of. Anyway, I was being too pessimistic, sniffing trouble where only a threat of it existed and imputing to Coralie motives that she probably didn't have. The reason she hadn't turned up at the clinic was maybe due to her getting fed up with Oliver.

When the door opened I jumped. It was Wynn, dazzling in a blue dress so pale it was almost ice. Enormous eyes flashing, naughty black stockings and a gold chain around one ankle, she strode to Barney and straightened his bedclothes.

As she bent over him he winked at me and said, 'They're real. None of your falsies here I can assure you.'

'Get on with you, Mr O.,' said Mona giving him the evening paper she'd brought with her. 'He's such a pet,' she smiled at me on the way out.

'All the nurses competing to give you a bed bath!'

If it wasn't for Wynn, Barney said, if it wasn't for Wynn, he'd go batty altogether. She kept him going with her carry-on. That was it, Wynn's earthy approach and salty wit made her Barney's kind of woman. Tits and bums you got anywhere, I'd often heard him say, but humour in a woman wasn't that common and much to be prized when you found it, even though it took the gilt off the romantic gingerbread.

'We'll see what Mistress Mullen has to say about this . . .' I was interrupted by Frankie herself sweeping in. She laughed and asked, was I referring to the bold Mona?

The same, I said, knowing that Frankie wouldn't be jealous of Wynn. The type of woman Frankie couldn't stand was the dusty little ultra feminine woman who was always up early enough to get the biggest male worm.

'Did you bring me some scotch, Frankie?' Barney reared up eagerly. It was amazing, the amount of weight he'd lost in a few days.

'Shut up for God's sake, Carson would have a fit if he heard you. Wanting whisky after being snatched from the jaws of death?' Frankie stabbed at some hair that was falling over her face. She lunged forward to stop Barney yanking out his drip.

It was just when you wanted whisky, Barney moaned, lying here being subjected to ham-handed nurses doing undignified things to him. Forced to suffer the ministrations of crude and ignorant quacks who had no sensitivity or imagination. Everything was made worse because of his deafness Barney yelled. He was being taken advantage of in a heartless way. It struck me of course that Barney and myself had been chatting without his wearing his hearing aid, yet here he was trotting out his disability as a trump card again. But it was late, after nine, and I said I'd have to be going before I was thrown out.

'And they'd do it,' Barney grunted. 'There's a woman on here at nights who should have been an all-in wrestler!'

I slid out quickly before the storm really burst but Frankie raced after me. I braced myself for an onslaught about the ingratitude of Barney, but all she said was:

'It's great to see Osborne riding again isn't it, Joyce? He must have the most terrific resilience to bounce back so quickly. Listen, I hate telling you this, but I think you ought to know. As I was coming here this evening I saw Oliver talking to Coralie Kane outside Robsons the jewellers.'

It must, must, be a mistake, I said. Frankie had never seen Coralie after all. And Oliver would never be daft enough to have anything to do with Mrs Kane after I'd told him to keep away. It couldn't be Coralie . . .

'Platinum hair? Curvy?' Frankie went on to make a figure of eight with her hands and I felt the knot of apprehension forming in my guts.

'I can't do any more,' I groaned. 'If Oliver insists on going in up to his neck then none of us can save that neck.'

'No,' said Frankie. 'But be sure you don't get *your* neck on the block.'

'Any suggestions about what else I can do?'

'Have another go at Olwyn, that's what.'

I drove home feeling deadly. I'd almost rather work than try and fill in my half day which meant nothing but more time for worry. Only if I stayed in the hospital, it was on the cards I'd meet Oliver. Olwyn was at home making an apple tart with some fruit Charlie had brought her; she'd felt a bit queasy that morning and hadn't gone into work. That wasn't reassuring –she must have ultra-understanding bosses, I thought sourly, as she wiped her floury hands.

What was wrong, she asked, darting quick tense glances at me. She was wearing denims and a white T-shirt which made her seem absurdly young. Too young and vulnerable to have all this trouble about her damn fool of a husband I thought savagely, for I was getting tired and bone weary of the whole wretched business, the very worst feature of which was that I couldn't see an end except in débâcle.

'What is it, Joyce? It's about Oliver isn't it?' Olwyn had the same pinched, worn look she'd had when she had been telling me about her marriage. She produced cigarettes, lighting one with trembling clumsiness. 'I'd given it up, haven't smoked for two years,' she said with a fractured gaiety. Then added, 'It's about that Kane woman, isn't it? She's causing more trouble, isn't she?'

I was too depressed to prevaricate and I told her that yes, Oliver had been seeing Coralie, had even been seen talking to her in Yorkely.

Olwyn paled. Was I sure? Olwyn suddenly caught my hands. Her eyes were startlingly dark and bright, no pupils to be seen and all the lines that hid themselves when she was not worried were visible again. Her pallor was deathly.

'Give Oliver a chance, Joyce, please. Before he came here he was on the point of emigrating. He had an offer . . . it's still open . . . at a hospital in Christchurch, New Zealand. I don't want to go, I'm sure Oliver doesn't either. I want to stay here. To be settled, just for once. Not wandering all over the place . . . no roots . . . no place of our own . . .'

She'd talk to Oliver, she said, wiping her face. She wore no make-up so the handkerchief only made her look scrubbed and very young. My heart ached for her as she told me she'd speak to Oliver, get at him again, about being discreet. I must believe her, she pleaded, give them a last chance. She'd vouch for Oliver. Maybe he was only finishing up with Coralie Kane. He was so kind and he hated to hurt.

But a doctor, especially an experienced one, has no right to be so indiscreet, I thought, on my way out. Olwyn, in spite of her frailties, was the stronger partner, the one obviously who kept things together. But even she must find it hard to deal with her mercurial husband. Like mercury itself, he responded to heat by escalating and such intuition as I'd managed to garner over the years of working in hospital made me feel, almost smell, danger.

Chapter Thirteen

The next morning was exceptionally busy at the hospital. The phones rang without pause, almost every ward had an emergency and most of the junior doctors were in London sitting an examination. Poor Mrs Bell, knowing I wanted to leave early, did her best but even she couldn't sort out the problems which had arisen. When I was off the phone she told me that Oliver had been in the hospital since half past eight and that he was now putting up a drip in Gilbert Ward.

'You look a bit pale, Doctor. Listen, I'll tell anyone who rings that you're not well. And there's Doctor Stafford, he'll cope.'

Mrs Bell, admirable woman, was tact personified. She saw, she heard, she noticed, but unlike me she kept a guard on her tongue. She liked Oliver and had helped him with the paper work which can take up so much of a doctor's time, and she knew all the GPs, indeed she was quite an authority on their characters and abilities. She looked at me again and asked if I really felt all right. Did I need anything?

'I don't want to be rude,' she added quickly.

I said there was no need to apologise. But I knew Mrs Bell's question meant people were talking. She hoped there was no trouble? Doctor Stafford had seemed pre-occupied lately. She sat letting the question hang delicately. I decided to tell her what was bothering me because I was absolutely sure of her discretion and loyalty. Anyway she knew about Coralie because she said:

'It's that Kane woman bothering people again, isn't it? I know she's been writing letters to Doctor Stafford.'

'Did he answer them?'

'Sort of. Actually he let me do them and he signed them.'

That was all right then. Mrs Bell could be depended on to upset no apple-carts. I told her about Mrs Kane and her accusations, the letters to Mrs Stafford and the phone calls. Mrs Bell sighed and said it was all awful, most unfair because Doctor Stafford was so nice, such a good doctor, so good she'd been hoping that I'd be able to keep him on.

'That's it. Just the trouble,' I said grimly. 'What Oliver isn't good at is being discreet, especially just now when he's probationary as it were. How can I give him a reference . . . ?'

Again the telephone interrupted us. After a moment's listening Mrs Bell clapped a hand over the mouthpiece and said that it was Miss Pillsworth on the line and she wanted to talk to me about Wendy Cotton. Mrs Bell said she'd say I was out and to phone tomorrow, but I had to know about Wendy and why Kate Pillsworth was involved. That's all I needed, some of Kate's messing and interference. But she got her spoke in first and silenced me.

'Doctor Delaney. Please let me explain. I know you've been dealing with Mrs Cotton and I hope you won't mind my being assigned to the case.'

I nearly said I would if she was going to wreck the tenuous relationship I had with Wendy and alienate any rapport I had established. Then I *did* mind. Behave in fact, as she had with the Laceys. But the new, repentant Kate wasn't a myth or a flash in the pan. She apologised to me again and said she was trying her best to alter and hoped she wouldn't upset me.

'Not so much me as Wendy,' I said. The girl was traumatised and tremulous enough, I told Kate, and I would like her to come into hospital just as soon as she got the court case over.

'That's it. It is over,' Kate said. 'Wendy's been put on

probation and everything's suspended providing she has treatment. She is more than willing to accept this, so I was wondering when I could bring her in, Doctor?'

As soon as possible, there was a bed in Flower Ward for her and Doctor Stafford would see to her if she came this afternoon, I said.

'I suppose leopards *can* change their spots if they're young?' I said to Mrs Bell.

'Off you go, Doctor,' she replied, 'before you get involved again!'

And I went, cheered by Wendy's agreement to have treatment and Kate's new persona.

I didn't think I'd enjoy getting away from the hospital, yet as I drove off down the avenue I felt cares slip away. Miraculously, I forgot about the hospital and Oliver and had a lovely time wandering from shop to shop. I ate two cream cakes for my tea, bought a plant and some chocolates and treated and indulged myself with reckless abandon until I came to and realised it was nearly seven o'clock and I'd spent all my money. I hadn't much to show for it except the plant but I didn't care. Normally I'd feel as guilty as hell but this afternoon I rationalised by thinking that I'd needed the break and the spending spree. I understood why Mother, long ago, had always got a lift by buying a new hat.

I had to manoeuvre a bit to manage my parcels so I could get in the door to my flat. Olwyn suddenly appeared looking anxious. Christ, what was it now? I was anticipating doom as soon as I saw either of the Staffords. But Olwyn only wanted to tell me that she'd spoken to Oliver, done her best to warn him about keeping a clean slate if he wanted the job.

I was glad to hear it, I said, and something in my tone, the drag of my voice made Olwyn say solicitously:

'How tired you look, Joyce. I hope Oliver is a help to you. You must let him take more of the work over you know. He doesn't mind.'

It wasn't the work I said, although in truth, the amalgam of Sheena's trouble, Barney's collapse and the way Oliver had mismanaged Coralie was enough to dent anyone's armour. I looked at Olwyn.

How was Barney, she asked? Would it be all right if she went to visit him tonight? She hoped Oliver would come but you never knew what time he'd be back from the hospital. Barney, I said, was on the mend and as he was bored he'd be delighted to see Olwyn.

'But I warn you. He's crusty as hell. Everything's wrong. He's got over being grateful at being alive!'

'I bet he is though at bottom. Anyway, mustn't keep you, Joyce. I hope you have a good rest.'

But I didn't. I couldn't stop the thoughts churning in my mind. I was so uneasy that I phoned Frankie who had come back from seeing Barney.

'Bang on form,' she said. 'Moaning and groaning and giving out hell about hospital life. They've taken out his tube and removed the drips so he can eat normally. Of course he claims that he can't eat any of the slops as he calls them. I phoned Carson today and although he's pleased with Barney's progress he says he'll be in hospital for another two weeks. I must say I funked telling Barney. Let Carson do that himself. Wynn is a brick. I must give that girl some champagne though God knows she doesn't need any fizz. Oh, Olwyn came in just as I was going. She looks fine. I think everything is O.K. there, you know. Has to be. Oliver was probably being nice, going to meet Coralie.'

'Nice? I'd call it foolhardy. Listen, Frankie, I know her. You don't. She's like a tarantula, only nicely packaged on the outside.'

'Yes. From what I saw of her she's quite a dish if you like the Marilyn Monroe type.'

I felt apprehensive, I said, and had the distinct impression that Oliver thought I was just being a big bad wolf with almost an old maidish habit of seeing beds everywhere.

'That's exactly what you are doing, Joyce, if I may say so . . .'

Really, Frankie had no need to ask whether she should 'say so' because she always levelled with me where other people would prevaricate. She took me to task with her usual fluency. I must allow Oliver to get on with things. I was hovering too much, anticipating trouble before it happened. I was assuming anyway that Oliver wanted to stay in Barrington after his enquiry about the job but maybe he wanted to be on the move, his record showed that. But what about Olwyn, she'd said they wanted to stay hadn't she? Well, Olwyn was very nice, seemed to be a good wife in spite of what she'd told me. But then did we know her? Did we know anything about anybody when it came to it? Couples showed you what they wanted to show, not what was really happening. On and on she went until her silver tongue persuaded me that I must stop being a Jonah and try to cultivate a more healthy detachment from my work. I'd grumbled when I hadn't got an assistant and now here I was bewailing again. At the end of what Frankie called her 'spiff' I was almost grovelling at ever having mentioned Oliver and his problems.

So I must take a pull at myself and practise forgetting work when I left the hospital. Of course, she went on, it was easier for her because she had Barney who simply told her to shut up about her bloody patients and act more like a woman. Men were better at not feeling guilty, she added. I said humbly that I'd try and do what she said, wouldn't keep on about the Staffords. She was so right, I thought as I went and had a bath. I was becoming obsessed by them.

Fortunately for the next week I was too busy to give much thought or attention to the Staffords. Wendy came into hospital and within a few days she was calmer, a little more outgoing and prepared to consider living. She was delighted by Sheena's message of forgiveness and said she would love to meet her. The less I saw of Oliver the more I thought he was looking twitched and exhausted. His clay-white pallor had returned, his eyes were tragic and, if I hadn't made up my mind to try not to worry, I'd have been flung into another anxiety state. With my new hardness, I thought, let Olwyn worry, she's married to him and I'm not.

I saw Frankie only once because all her free time was spent with Barney who was still in St Basil's, but getting stronger and more vociferous daily. Full of jumping beans, Frankie said. She was planning a holiday break for herself and Barney at a palm court type of hotel where they could sit in the lounge being cosetted, exchanging comments about the other guests.

'You should come too, Joyce,' she said. 'We'll feel quite juvenile amongst the bath chairs and ear trumpets.'

I couldn't get time off at such short notice, I said. It was impossible. Even if I could, I wouldn't risk going to a hotel with Barney. But Frankie was elated, in top form now that he was restored to her, deafness and all, and she flung herself with her usual élan into preparation for the holiday.

Not that I couldn't do with a break. I was aware of being ratty and short-tempered and once or twice poor Mrs Bell looked reproachfully at me and I tried counting to ten, five anyway, before I spoke. Oliver continued to wilt and everyone now commented openly on how ill he looked.

Manners collared me one day and asked whether I knew if Oliver was applying for the vacant registrar's post, because he'd got three very suitable applicants, all with the right qualifications and one of them had passed the post-graduate examinations which Oliver hadn't attempted. I didn't know what was happening, I said, glad of a chance to air some doubts. Oliver, I thought, was interested and certainly his wife was. But I didn't know more than that and frankly, I added, feeling disloyal, I felt I couldn't do any more. I simply wasn't prepared to tackle Oliver. He was experienced and had been qualified long enough to know his own mind for God's sake.

Manners looked at me sharply. 'Do I detect disenchantment with the wonder boy?' he quizzed. 'He's a right rolling stone and no mistake,' he went on, 'I don't think he wants to settle you know. Blotted too many copy-books I'd say. You get these high-flyers, you know, great on fancy diagnoses and impressing the nurses, but short on commonsense. You see, they've made the entry to medical school so blocked with IQ and high A levels that the academic whizz kids are the only ones, on the whole, that are able to get into medical school. But there's no real estimate of sense and sensibility. Everyone knocks the old way with its closed shop entry and emphasis on a family connection with medicine. But the Old Boy network *did* mean you knew what you were getting and if a rotter did slip through the net, then the ranks closed and the situation or the body was dealt with, behind closed doors. Scandal was avoided. In Stafford's situation, ten or fifteen years ago, he'd be hauled before the Medical Superintendent and given a roasting and a warning. Now there's a great big nothing. Nobody with the power to sack so no one takes responsibility.'

Anyway, I said, Oliver was only a locum and could be got rid of any time. I couldn't help feeling a sneaky relief that he hadn't applied for the job and thus let me off the hook as regards a reference. But even if Oliver *did* apply now, and there was one day to go before the closing date for applications, I was sure that he wouldn't be short-listed. I knew by Manners's words that he didn't want Oliver to stay, even as a locum.

I tried not to start my cycle of fears again and dashed off, because I had to visit a man who had become maniacal in the past week and whose wife was so worn out that she kept telephoning the police. The call sounded urgent so I decided to skip lunch and I phoned Oliver and asked him to start my clinic because I thought I would be late. Oliver said that Mr Latimer wanted to talk to me.

'Doctor. I thought you'd be coming to Gilbert this morning,' He was speaking so quietly I could hardly hear. 'Have to keep me voice down because Doctor Stafford's here. Now you know how I dislike calling doctors. Never had to do this before but I'm worried about Doctor Stafford. He's not well, Doctor. He filled the ECT syringes with the wrong stuff this morning and he arrived on the ward before eight. He looks far from well . . . far from well. Even the patients are talking.'

When there is risk to patients then action is called for. And Latimer was prissy in manner but shrewd enough in his comments, and his devotion to the patients was a legend in the hospital. I thanked him for telling me and I knew that I wasn't off any hook, I was impaled, responsible and I had to deal with Stafford. It would have to be after the clinic.

The domiciliary call to Mr Ernie Tickle, the manic patient, took me two hours because he was in that most difficult mental state which makes someone feel that they can do anything and go anywhere. All reason goes, or is blunted, and the patient feels super-charged, mental cylinders blasting. To manics like the unfortunate Mr Tickle normal people seem to be simply obstructive. Ernie was like Mrs Ainsworth without the regal delusions.

It had taken ages for someone to answer the door of the Tickle's house and I was on the point of going away in defeat when Mrs Tickle appeared looking tired and raddled. She'd been up every night for a week with her husband. He refused to see the doctor, had banished a social worker and threatened her with eviction unless she stopped annoying him. She was sure he wouldn't see me and even if he did he'd just be rude, she went on. Or else run off the way he had when Doctor Mason called yesterday. Her poor eyes were watery all the time and she looked as if she needed hospitalisation herself. She had angina, was supposed to rest, she said, but if she left Ernie alone, he'd either get run over by a car when he dashed out, or start badgering the neighbours. Already the woman next door was fit to be tied because Ernie had rushed in the morning before and harangued the neighbour's octogenarian father who, as a result, had to be sent to hospital after suffering a stroke brought on by being frightened by Ernie.

'He's trampling around upstairs,' Mrs Tickle said trembling. 'Listen to him talking away. That's what I have night and day. One of my sons tries to come nights but he's working shifts and it's not easy. Something will have to be done, Doctor, else I'll break down meself I will. There's no knowing what he'll do when he's like this. He was in Barrington Hall six years ago under Doctor Manners and he put him on Lenium . . . I mean Lilium . . .'

Lithium, I said. People prone to mania and depression are stabilised on this long-acting drug now, as a prophylaxis against an attack rather than a treatment. The trouble was, as I well knew, that when people began to become disturbed again they lost insight and didn't bother to take their Lithium because, like Mr Tickle, they imagined that they had never felt better in their lives.

'He's in a dreadful state,' poor Mrs Tickle wept. 'He's that particular when he's well, never out of the bathroom. This morning he . . . he . . . well, he drank his own urine saying that it was good for him.'

'And so it is. Best treatment there is,' said a wiry little man who appeared down the stairs. Bald, with a dirty vest and long baggy underpants, he was, he announced, going jogging.

'But this lady's come to see you, Ernie. To try and help you . . .' Mrs Tickle said nervously.

Her husband, bloodshot eyes glittering and mouth cracked from malnutrition, said that he needed no help, drinking his water was keeping him going. That and jogging.

From his wasted appearance and greyish pallor I'd bet Mr Tickle was barely able to stand up leave alone jog. What with his age, his disturbed mental state and lack of nourishment I could see something had to be done quickly. No use arguing or reasoning with a mania this advanced. Mr Tickle said that he couldn't delay, he was wasting time talking to us and indeed he shoved past us and set off down the path, withered bottom waggling in the absurd way old runners and milers sometimes have of twisting their bodies. Elbows stuck out like needles and bald head down he was off down the road.

A woman, swollen body and thin frightened face, wiped her floury hands on her overall and called from the next doorway that Ernie would do himself in, drop dead, and that something ought to be done. He should be put away, she went on fixing me with a ferocious look. I was used to that. Used to having people talk lightly about other people 'being put away'. It wasn't that easy, I explained to Mrs Tickle. Certainly her husband had to go to hospital so that he could be calmed down and treated. As it was patently clear he wouldn't go willingly I'd have to 'commit' him, which I proposed to do. But the documents needed the social worker's recommendation and the signature of the GP. I'd do my part, get Social Services and set things up for admission to Barrington. Had she a phone? Not that I'd be able to get a social worker to come right away. It was still lunch time after all.

'In here, Doctor . . .' Mrs Tickle showed me into the front parlour, stuffy and fusty with photographs of the family in violent colours everywhere. As I phoned I was riveted by a wedding photograph of the Tickles. Ernie had wavy hair plastered all over his forehead and was so fat he was bursting out of his demob suit, while Mrs Tickle was all teeth and eyes on a tailored costume. I stared at the photograph for several minutes as I tried to get someone to take a message for Rod Butler, the social worker for the area in which the Tickles lived. They were all out the girl said, but could she take a message? It would have to be, I said, because I had to rush back to a clinic but would she emphasise that it was urgent and should be seen today? It was her job to convey messages accurately, she said stiffly, and I apologised. God, I seemed to do nothing but upset people these days, I thought wearily, putting the phone down.

'They had this trouble last time,' Mrs Tickle said, her handkerchief to her mouth. 'Every time someone came Ernie would go out. Like he has now. And I can't go through another night like last. He keeps some swords, that's his hobby, collecting military swords, see, and when he's like this he has a habit of taking 'em down and waving 'em at me. And going on and on about Burma and that. Right enough, they thought highly of him in the army and he's got some medals and that. But I don't fancy him waving the swords about again. Especially as me son can't get tonight . . .'

She had no need to worry, I said. The vision of Mr Tickle and swords was pretty frightening, but the wheels were in motion and even if Mr Tickle didn't come back, Social Services would ensure that he'd be found eventually. She wouldn't be left on her own to cope.

'I'm very grateful to you,' she said.

Her old eyes watered with continual tears, some obstruction in the tear ducts I thought, and she had a sort of tic which made her head veer sharply to one side. She smelled of camphor and body sweat and the onions she must have eaten in the past day or two. Would I have some tea? Or coffee? I was glad that I had the excuse of my clinic. The vision of Mr Tickle drinking his urine wasn't pleasant.

I had a shock when I found that it was after four o'clock, five by the time I reached the hospital where I got a greater shock. There were no patients there, no one except Coralie

Kane, sitting up primly in another new creation of turquoise linen. Hair in its usual pale perfection and a tight smile that I didn't like at all.

Morgan rushed up to me looking anxious and worried. 'Something's up, Doctor. I think it's to do with Mrs Kane. Doctor Stafford wants to see you.'

It was like the nightmare becoming the actuality. I felt the familiar liquidation in my limbs, the horrible inability to move, always experienced when I had a bad dream of the enemy appearing over the hill, the SS about to storm my house and the barbarians at the gate.

'I got through the patients,' Oliver looked ashen. 'Knew you were held up. But there's some bad news I'm afraid.'

Tell me, for God's sake tell me, was it to do with Mrs Kane waiting outside? I slumped down in a chair, bracing myself, anticipating disaster. And it came.

Oliver spoke slowly, heavily, as if he felt unreal, too, was also going through some bizarre and macabre dance which would be over soon. Meantime, both of us felt displaced and detached, almost whirled around in some poisoned fantasy which would slow and wind down just as we might come out of anaethesia and hear 'cough please'. Meantime, there was no antidote. 'I'm sorry, Joyce. The fact is that Coralie is threatening to write to the GMC about me. Claiming that I . . . that I wanted sex with her and that the reason I was stopped from seeing her is because she refused.'

It wasn't worth even hinting at 'I told you so'. Too late to learn, to threaten even, I'd done that already. I was bursting with an impotent rage against Stafford. Trailing his indiscretions after him like a turd left on a carpet. It wasn't as if he didn't know, as if I hadn't begged him to lay off. I was afraid to say anything or I would, I was sure, lose all control and become a shrilling fish wife of invective and vituper-ation. There he sat, shaken, ashen, hang-dog. His bloody 'little boy lost' air again. Well, he was well and truly lost now.

'Frankie saw you the other night, when you met Coralie, after I expressly told you not to,' I told him.

'She was blackmailing. Threatening. I thought I could talk her out of it.'

'Does Olwyn know?'

'Not yet. I'll tell her tonight. Unless you could have a word with her first.'

That did it. The cool assumption that I might do his dirty work was more than I could stand. He was more than a fool, I said, he was a craven one and even his record of being a top class clinician wouldn't save him from the high jump. He was finished in Barrington, I didn't even bother to tell him about what Manners said about the job. Olwyn would have to be told as soon as possible. I'd leave that to him. What was now in jeopardy was his professional reputation. The maintenance of his name on the medical register. I nearly tore myself asunder trying to keep calm.

Morgan, who came in with a tray of tea, looked at Stafford and myself, with her lips working as if she was chewing gum, a habit she had when she was worried.

'I presume,' I said handing him tea, 'I presume you're a member of one of the defence societies?' Fees were going up annually but no doctor neglected payment because litigation was increasing, especially among patients like Coralie Kane. Just like a reckless psychopath of Oliver's ilk not to be a member though. But he said, yes, that he was.

Anger, the first flames of it anyway, was waning. I can never sustain aggression at boiling point. No virtue in that really because fury makes me feel sick. Now, I was beginning to be conscious of a weary, blank sort of acceptance, almost a relief that my deep-seated hunch was proved right. It had been like a collection of pus which couldn't be incised and therefore treated until the time of ripening, a time which old medical text books used to refer to as 'the time of election'.

But maybe I didn't know the worst. 'What exactly is Coralie saying? Or threatening to report?'

'As I said. That I made "suggestions" . . .' His voice trailed off.

Maybe he thought I wanted to probe. I did not. The danger was not what he did or didn't do but that he had made a dangerous association with a patient. The old school girl tag 'an occasion of sin' flashed foolishly through my mind. 'It has to be more than that,' I said. Coralie wasn't that much of a mug, if it came to accusations of rape then her file was crammed with the history of her allegations. Which Stafford should have read. 'What's she saying?' I asked.

He sat hunched in his chair like a patient. 'What she's saying is that I called to see her one evening after the clinic. A man friend of hers was hiding and is saying that he saw me. That I spent two hours there.'

So that was it. The old, old story chewed up every week by one of the Sunday papers. I could see the headlines now. 'Blonde accuses sex mad doctor.' 'Home visit becomes orgy.' And then the complaint to the GMC. In which I would have to be involved because Oliver worked for me. I couldn't think properly, only anticipate and imagine the trouble which was only a small fire at the moment, but knowing Coralie's venom, I had no doubt that it could become a blazing furnace.

'Let me try and get it straight. Coralie is threatening to complain to the GMC that you've been unprofessional. She has a witness to prove that you were visiting her at home on a certain night . . .'

I paused because I couldn't believe that a doctor could do anything so senselessly reckless as to call on an out-patient attending his clinic for no particular purpose. Oh yes, maybe there was purpose, I was beginning to learn just how insanely imprudent Oliver was. After all, if he met Coralie openly in Yorkely, and that was fact, he'd be capable of anything wouldn't he?

'Of course I didn't go to her home. She's lying. I should have listened to you when you warned me. I'm awfully sorry, truly . . .'

'Shut up,' I rasped. I was trying to marshal my thoughts, to bring some sort of order to a nightmare which had become reality. Coralie had a witness. Had Oliver an alibi? With almost uncanny intuition Oliver seemed visibly to pull himself together.

'I was visiting Barney. Mona Wynn was there, too, and just coming off duty, so we went for a drink. She was telling me all about a management course she was thinking of going on.'

This shred of hope galvanised me and my mind began to work again, collating the data. Whether Oliver was with Mona or not was beside the point; I was too desperate to spend time in assessing whether she was merely a last minute invention of Oliver's.

'She'd be prepared to back you up? Stand by you?' I asked and he nodded.

'Of course. She owes me a few favours,' he said, in a brief return of his maddening confidence.

'I hope you're right.'

I felt the beat of a starting migraine and I rooted in my bag for some aspirin. My mouth was dry and I chewed the tablet because I couldn't swallow it and then I almost gagged with the bitter taste of the powder. Had he any idea why Coralie wanted to see me? It was a silly question in truth. Coralie wanted, of course, to give herself the supreme satisfaction of delivering what she no doubt hoped would be an incendiary bomb. He supposed she wanted to tell me about all this, Oliver said miserably. He'd known about it for some time but hoped he could stall her, deflect her paranoid obsession with doctors and their failings.

'But you know what she's like,' he said. 'I thought I was beginning to help her, that I was about to stumble across what's really bugging her and getting her to come to terms with herself, able to face life and all its problems.'

After all, Oliver's drive to help others was that same therapeutic impulse which had resulted in the finding of Melinda. It was unfortunate that that same zeal had been misdirected in Coralie's case and I couldn't stop thinking about my own responsibility in handing over a hot potato like Coralie to a doctor who was, when it came down to it, a junior in status. It was my clinic, the patients were my patients and I was the responsible Medical Officer in law.

The aspirin was starting to work and my head had stopped the premonitory throbbing which heralded migraine. I swallowed some water because the adrenalin which must be coursing through my system was making my mouth arid and I could feel sweat trickling wetly down my back. Had I got it straight? I asked, looking at Oliver who had got up from the chair he'd slumped on and was now pacing up and down, hands stuffed in his pockets. His hair was spiky, like an enlarged wire dish cleaner, and the dark eyes were flickering under my gaze, like a patient with the unco-ordinated eye movements that are called 'nystagmus'. What the hell sort of an impression would he make on an austere body of medical colleagues like the General Medical Council? With his almost gawping expression and baggy black suit he looked like a clerk caught in a shady act like rifling the till.

'You tell me that nothing improper happened between you and Mrs Kane, that you didn't call at her house and at the time she claims you visited her you were in fact with Nurse Wynn.'

'That's it.' Oliver said eagerly. 'I did accept the odd present from her,' he added looking at me sideways.

'Like what?' Blast him. Just as I was beginning to think that perhaps everything would fizzle out and that even if it didn't Oliver had Mona to support him.

'Just cigarettes from time to time. Oh yes, she did bring me a cake she made once. I thought it would be good treatment to accept the odd thing from her, that it would make her feel a bit more normal and as if she mattered in the clinical transaction. I didn't see anything wrong in that, honestly I still don't. I really thought I was helping her, Joyce. I know you don't like her and I don't know why she's having a go like this, but all I can say is that I gave her a tremendous amount of time because I was sorry for her and thought I could help her cope with her problems.'

Just as well try and teach a piranha fish to give up meat, I thought wearily. Now we had to see Coralie and I hoped, squash her. But when she tripped in and arranged herself on the chair in front of me I had a paralysing conviction that nothing would make her relinquish the lime-light. After all, this bombshell she proposed to throw was a marvellous opportunity to try and destroy some of the hated band of doctors whom she loathed but still couldn't keep away from.

'Well, Coralie.' I studied her, conscious of Oliver hovering behind me.

Coralie threw him a withering glance which had a certain heavy flirtatiousness in it. She was wearing a baby-blue dress and her pile of newly blonded hair was lint white. There was a strong smell of torrid gardenia perfume and I noticed that her eye shadow had been carefully selected to tone perfectly with her dress. She patted her hair with one hand, boneless, white and dimpled. 'Of course, you weren't going to see me again, were you, Doctor Delaney? But now of course you've got to, haven't you? Sitting out there waiting, I bet my cheeks should be burning the way you've been discussing me.' Her coral lips parted to reveal small pearly teeth which looked false, but were in fact her own. She'd often told me that her teeth, eyes, and ears were the only parts of her body which worked properly. 'You see . . .' she said, 'People don't believe me. That makes me cross. Very cross. After all, I'm a poor, lonely woman struggling to keep going. I need help and I don't get it. Specially from people who *should* help me, like doctors.'

Come on, spit it out, cut the cackle and the nauseating innuendos, I wanted to shout at her. But instead I made my voice as professionally steady as I could and asked why she was here and what I could do for her. Her pale imitation of a smile appeared again and she giggled, a titter that was as free of warmth as her smile.

'It's not for you to do anythin', Doctor Delaney,' she smirked. 'It's what I'm going to do.'

Chapter Fourteen

The stench of Coralie's perfume, the sight of her, like some rank weed breeding with venomous fertility, made me want to make a rush at her and shake her out of her poisonous complacency. What did she want, I asked again.

'What do I want?' She preened and shoved out that misleading soft bosom. 'Better ask *him*.' She nodded towards Oliver.

'I've already spoken to Doctor Stafford and he's given me his account of what happened. Now it's your turn. We're both listening. Come on, Coralie, you're making allegations against Doctor Stafford. What are they?' I asked.

'Only that he propositioned me several times. Wanted sex with me, if you want it crudely. And he called at my house. Which I can prove because I've got a witness, a friend who saw him come and timed when he left, so it's no use you doctors sticking together and trying to hush this up.' The last shot was delivered with an angry toss of her massive pompadour.

She was seriously suggesting that Doctor Stafford had behaved improperly to her, I asked again.

'I'm not *suggesting* anything,' she hissed. 'I'm telling you, telling you that Stafford's a filthy beast. He wants reporting, a man like him, in his position.'

She glared at Oliver who had stopped his pacing and was staring at her. Why didn't he jump up and repudiate what Coralie was saying? Now she was talking about how her trust in him had been misplaced: oh yes, he'd been good to her at first, really helped her, until he started asking her to stay when patients had left the clinic and then there were his demands.

'The same rotten game that other men play with me,' she spat. 'Just when I was, like he called it, "having a healthy relationship at last".'

Paranoid, yes. But so pat and convincing that I'd swear she'd practised this at home. Her eyes gleamed with tears and she used a tiny lace handkerchief with all the skill of her undoubted acting ability. What the hell was Oliver thinking about?

I rallied myself and said, 'Do you realise what you're saying, Coralie? The seriousness of your allegations?'

'Course I do. But people like him should be shown up.'

'Doctor Stafford denies everything,' I said and she laughed again, a mirthless squeak.

'Well, he would, wouldn't he? But I have proof. And I know where to send it. I found out about the General Medical Council and how they can stop doctors working, take them off the register.'

I began to feel frightened suddenly. Oliver could produce an alibi, sure enough, but even so, no doctor can avoid the enquiry which must follow an allegation, however vicious, if it is made in the proper form, and the mud is bound to stick somewhere. Why didn't he say something? Christ, it could be, it just could be, that Coralie was speaking the truth. I felt the lack of fear. 'You have a right to complain,' I said sharply. 'Any patient has in the National Health, but you'd better be able to substantiate what you say, otherwise Doctor Stafford can have you for libel and slander.'

'Tell me something I don't know, will you? I've complained often enough, haven't I? And been ignored and made to feel like I was dirt. But this time they'll listen won't they? Or so my solicitor says.'

Her malicious grin had all the spite in the world in it and I thought, God, she's got Oliver by the shortest of hairs. He must have thought so, too, because he seemed to come to life, to jerk himself out of his shocked silence.

'Now it's my turn,' he said. 'I've listened to you, Coralie.

trying to make sense of what you're talking about. Why are you doing this? What for?' There was real agony in his voice, and Coralie looked away. 'You know I've done my best for you,' he went on. 'I've done everything possible to make you feel better. And yet you come here to put out all those lies about me. I just don't understand.' He threw his arms out in a beseeching way. He just could not manufacture such pain. For a ghastly few seconds I thought he was going to cry, the way his face quivered and his voice trembled.

Coralie stared at him expressionlessly and then she said, 'I'm sticking to what I said. And it happened the way I said it, too.'

'You asked me to visit, many times, sure. But I have always refused. Explained to you so many times why I couldn't call to your house and tried to give you extra time here at the clinic.'

Coralie's face cracked into another malevolent smile. 'I want to stop other women being molested by doctors like you,' she said, her tone virtuous, her false concern unctuous. I could have slung something at her, the second time she'd brought out the beast in me this evening. I heard Oliver make a noise, it was the drop of his stethoscope on the floor and as he bent to pick it up Coralie smirked.

'You won't be using that after the GMC have done with you, will you?'

Patients often used terms like 'something snapped'. I could almost hear the crack of Oliver's inner reserve. His head lunged forward like an outraged tortoise and his voice was electric with fury. Maybe it was the sight of Coralie so coldly triumphant or the sight of the stethoscope which symbolised his job. Whatever the reason he abandoned his air of stunned martyrdom and lashed out at Coralie. 'You must,' he said, 'be much sicker than I thought, to hate me like this and want to destroy me.'

His eyes were black pools of fury and his white face had broken into small rivers of sweat. I'd never ever seen him show aggression leave alone this black and bitter anger. He's innocent, he's got to be, no man could act this well, I thought, as Coralie began to whimper and say that it was no good him trying to bully her, that she was going on with her complaint and he'd not stop her. Him or anyone else, she added, giving me a smouldering look.

'Then bloody go ahead.' Oliver shouted. There was such maddened pain in the way he was now leaning on the table, bending forward as if to prevent himself falling to pieces that even Coralie smelled of fear.

She gathered herself up, wobbling slightly on her steepled heels. The gardenia scent was diluted by her sweat. We were all roused in a primitive way, our hormones pumping out the adrenalin of fear in response to danger.

Oliver straightened and made a move towards Coralie. She must have thought, as I did, that he was going to strike her because she gave a yelp and dashed to the door. 'Go on. Do what you like. I don't bloody care,' Oliver shouted.

Coralie paused, obviously searching for a parting shot. She opened her mouth like an expectant fish but said nothing. We sat and listened to the clack of her disappearing heels.

'Wow! Sorry about that. It's only the second time in my life that I've let fly, lost my temper.' Oliver sat down, the anger still giving an edge to his voice and his eyes still dark with fury. 'She's everything you said she was. Everything. She really wants to ruin me!'

Pity you didn't listen to what I said about her, I was thinking, but aloud I said that 'ruin' was going too far and after all he had his alibi with Mona, hadn't he? . . . Or had he? For a terrifying moment I played again with the possibility of this being a lie.

'Yes. Mona will stand by me, no worry about that. It's just that I don't want her to be involved and get bad publicity herself. And there's Olwyn. Christ, I'll have to tell her.'

'I hate to say it, but that's your problem, Oliver. Listen, let's go over it again. You saw Coralie here at the clinic, sometimes on her own. She gave you some small presents which you accepted. But you never called to her house and on the night she says that you did call you were having a drink with Mona Wynn who's prepared to stand by you. O.K.?'

Oliver was standing, hands in pockets, staring miserably at the wall in front of him. Then he looked straight at me and said quietly, 'No more than that. But I suppose the GMC will take the view that I should have had a chaperone if I did see Coralie on her own. They'll take a poor view of my not twigging how dangerous she was, is.'

We'd have to hope things didn't reach the stage of getting to the GMC, I said.

Coralie was obviously hell bent on squeezing the maximum attention from a situation, so floridly dramatic that it must be the answer to her prayers for the notice which she felt had always been denied her. After all, the situation had all the ingredients for scandal.

'I'm terribly sorry dragging you into this, Joyce. But, please, please believe me. I haven't done what she's accusing me of. Honest.'

I believed him, I said. I had to, I thought to myself. The alternative couldn't be borne. I tried to pull my scattered wits together. Coralie didn't know Oliver had an alibi. At this stage it might be wise not to tell her. Anyway she'd dashed out before we had the chance. The phone interrupted my thoughts. It was the hospital. They'd been trying to bleep me but my bleep mustn't be working. Oh God, I'd forgotten I was on duty.

'Doctor Drummond here, Doctor Delaney. I don't know whether you can help at all. I've got this family on my list, the Foleys. They're a problem family in every way. The father's just out of prison for GBH, Grievous Bodily Harm, the mother's pregnant with her sixth and two of the sons are in Borstal. Oh . . . and one of the daughters has taken up with a Jamaican who beats her. You get the picture?'

Yes, indeed. It was the sort of situation I could have done without. There wasn't much I could do, that was for sure, and I felt so tired and hot and generally worried, that coping with the Foley clan was the last thing I wanted. But Drummond was kind and caring and rarely asked Barrington for help. He said again that he knew there was little I could do but the family kept phoning him, Social Services, everybody indeed other than the police. I guessed he was asking for a visit as a last and despairing hope.

My watch said seven o'clock, I'd visit the Foleys in about an hour's time after I'd had a bath and changed. No good trying to figure out strategy for Oliver till I was less tired and clearer in my head. He must have felt the same because he didn't speak on the way back in the car with me to the Priest's House. Perhaps he was thinking about how to tell Olwyn. Then it struck me that he should wait, till tomorrow anyway. He greeted this suggestion with some relief and added rather hopelessly that maybe we could sort something out between us.

I had a bath and was just making myself a pot of tea when Frankie rang.

She'd been thinking, she said, in that slightly breathless way she had when she'd had a good idea. Barney was home, did I know that? Before I could say how pleased I was she galloped on; Barney was a wee bit bored and so she was going to have a few people over tomorrow night. Just me and the Staffords and Mona Wynn; we could help eat the enormous salmon one of her patients had given her. Lovely, I said cautiously, I felt more like a wake than a party I thought inside. Yes, it was a marvellous idea, I went on, but the notice was a bit short. Nonsense, she said briskly and I knew it was no good arguing. I hadn't the energy to do so anyway. Olwyn and Mona had accepted, Frankie said, and she'd see me tomorrow night, about eight.

'Listen, Frankie. There's a bit of trouble. No. I can't tell you now. I'll phone you tomorrow.' Before her curiosity could overcome my reticence I slammed down the receiver after telling her that, yes, I'd come over to Garland House tomorrow night.

It was only after two hours spent with the Foleys in their dilapidated house in misnamed Lovely Lane that I remembered the business of Oliver. Like some rotten tooth whose nerve was exposed to a blast of heat, the twinge of worry renewed itself; at least the Foleys had served as a counter-irritant.

I said to Mr Foley that I was very sorry I couldn't do anything, and Mr Foley, with the resignation born of too many defeats, said that he understood. But Serena, their daughter, too young to have grown used to failure, looked up from chucking her fat black baby under the chin and asked me whether I could stop her drunken and aggressive husband from his boozy battering at the front door. What about the police? I asked.

She made a face and said hopelessly, 'They can't do nuthin', they say, less I get a junction or something.'

Yes, I thought, and even if she did get an injunction, the police wouldn't want to know.

'Doctor . . .' Mrs Foley had come to the door with me. She stared at me and said, 'Maybe you *can* do something. Not make our troubles go away, like – but couldn't you put us all on some pills to help us put up with them?'

Ah, the happy pills I didn't have. If I had I'd take them myself, I said gently.

Chapter Fifteen

When I returned from the Foley visit I tried to think over the facts facing Oliver and myself and to come up with a solution to deal with them. The more I grappled with the sordid affair the less I could come to a plan of campaign. So I decided to copy Scarlett O'Hara and leave the worry till the morning. That didn't work either because sleep evaded me, so I got up at seven o'clock and was just pouring out my third cup of coffee when the phone went. It was Frankie.

'What's up? Tell me all about it. I'll be on the move so much this morning, and this afternoon I've got to have my hair done. So spit it out. It's Oliver, isn't it?' she asked.

'Why do you say that? Have you heard anything?' It was close shooting on Frankie's part right enough.

'Come on, you're speaking to another hardened professional, Joyce. No, it's just that we still don't know much about him and he's got a sort of doomed quality about him And of course, it's on the cards that trouble has prevented him going further in his career. Tell me all about it.'

So I told her and as always she was an excellent person to chew the cud with. She listened. You didn't have to repeat things to her and, like me, Coralie infuriated her.

'Nasty little cow,' she said. 'But how bloody stupid of Oliver to see her alone. Listen, you don't think it's true, what she's saying do you?'

'Oliver says no, and he's got an alibi with Mona Wynn,' I told her. 'Says he was with her that night.'

'That's something anyway because Mona will stand firm. Oh God, what a mess. Is there any chance Kane will retract?' Frankie asked.

'Not at all,' I said. 'Far from retracting, Coralie's enjoying every bit of juice she can extract from the whole wretched affair. I can't see a way out,' I added gloomily.

After we'd spoken to each other for all of half an hour we'd only got to the stage of wondering whether, if the worst came to the worst, we could maybe organise a round robin of loyalty from some of Oliver's patients.

'God, I must go,' Frankie concluded, 'I can hear Barney thumping about.'

Me too, I said. Did she really expect us all tonight? Of course, Frankie said, we could have a council of war over the salmon. Then she asked whether Olwyn knew about things. No, I said, that was another nasty chore we had to do, or at least Oliver had to do; I'd advised him to leave that till today was over, anyway.

Then just as I was about to fling on my clothes a 'eureka' flash hit me. Mona Wynn! Mona Wynn! Suppose, just suppose, she could be persuaded to confront Coralie with the thing that Coralie didn't know, that Oliver had been with her on the night of the 'visit'? I sat down and thought hard. Yes, the ploy was suddenly obvious, but full of difficulties and there was no time to spare. Mona might be away or not willing to beard Coralie, or Coralie mightn't be in.

I jumped up and dashed to the phone. I knew Mona worked days and when the young student nurse who answered the call to St Basil's said that Nurse Wynn was going temporary night duty I could have screamed with frustration.

'But I can give you her flat number.' The nurse sounded a nice child. 'You could try there during the day and of course she comes on duty at eight o'clock this evening.'

I took the number and thought. My plan couldn't wait till tonight when Mona would be on duty anyway. So I dialled her flat number but there was no reply. Perhaps Mona was in transit. I'd try from the hospital.

I grabbed my bag and rushed out just in time to see

Olwyn coming out of the front door. She looked different, not so fresh, and her eyes were puffy. God, maybe Oliver has told her, I thought; she looks as if she's been crying. I didn't want to see her, I dreaded what she was going to say but she latched on to me eagerly.

'Gorgeous morning isn't it?' she said brightly.

No, she couldn't know. I sensed that, because in spite of her rather puffy eyes and the pallor which wasn't her usual alabaster, there was the touch of what Frankie had said without seeing her, a 'suet pudding'.

'The morning's lovely but I'm late,' I said edging to my car. But Olwyn paused and looked around her, the front of the Priest's House was dark with old trees but today the sun was so hot and piercing that Olwyn and I had to shade our eyes.

'Look Olwyn,' I said hastily, 'I've got to rush, love. I'll see you tonight. At Frankie's.' But she wanted to tell me something, she said, smiling brilliantly at Charlie who was passing us with the post. Before I could brace myself for what I was positive Olwyn was going to come out with, she smiled, another almost foolishly delighted grin.

'I've been sick,' she said. 'Isn't it great? I must tell someone, Joyce. I'm pregnant, Joyce. And I'm so happy about it . . .' She flung her arms out in a gesture so spontaneously joyous that I couldn't help feeling joy with her.

Did Oliver know? I asked. A nasty thought jarred me, was the baby Oliver's? But her next words made me castigate myself for unworthiness.

'We've waited so long, wanted a baby so badly that we were afraid to hope. And this is Oliver's baby, the best present I could give him. I'm so very happy. I'd have told Oliver last night but he looked so worried and tired. Is everything all right, Joyce? In the hospital?'

So I lied as diligently as I could to her, told her I was so pleased for her, just as I was sure Oliver would be. Another thing, she said, they'd been talking about that job in New

Zealand, the salary was so good, she was certain that now with the baby coming they'd take it and, she added happily, that things were at last working out for them. Everything, even a new life, was opening up. Yes, yes, I lied, this really seemed so.

As she walked, no tripped, away down the road I got into my car and drove in misery to the hospital. The only thing was that I did at least have a plan and till it failed we would keep things from Olwyn. She had told me, before we parted, that she was going to tell Oliver about her pregnancy when we were at Frankie's.

There was still Mona to be contacted. Before I started the day's work I dashed into a small office used by the dentist on his weekly visit to the hospital and I phoned Mona again. The phone rang and rang and then there was Mona's voice. She sounded so sleepy, almost slurred.

'I had a hellish night,' she said, and I felt dreadful when she apologised for, as she put it, 'sounding drunk'. But she'd dropped off to sleep in her clothes. 'Didn't even make the bed,' she said. I in turn apologised frantically and asked whether she knew about Mrs Kane's allegations. She said she didn't and then her voice sharpened, came alive. She was all shocked attention when I told her what Coralie proposed doing.

'But she can't. She can't do anything. Oliver was with me on that night,' she said.

I asked her whether she was prepared to stand by this? In public? And in writing?

'Need you ask?' Her tone sounded hurt. 'Oliver's a smashing doctor,' she went on, 'and I'm very fond of Olwyn. Of course I'll do anything to help, anything. But what?'

I told her what I wanted her to do, to go down to Coralie, confront her with Oliver's alibi, and maybe, just maybe, she'd retract.

There was silence and I thought, Christ, she's not going to play ball, she's wanting out of the whole messy business, understandable with her being so totally dependant on her job. It wasn't fair to ask her to involve herself in the slime of a scandal which, if it blew up as Coralie meant it to, held many brickbats and no bouquets. Despairingly, I told her of Olwyn's pregnancy.

'Of course I'll do what you ask; you don't have to sell it. I was just thinking how we go about it,' Mona said crisply. 'I'd like to see this Kane woman and well, if not having a go at her, though I'd like to, confront her with our closed ranks. Yes, I'm on. What about times and that?'

I told Mona how to get to Coralie's. Mona said she'd have to have some sleep first because she wanted all her wits about her to deal with Coralie, not to be zombified, the way she was now. She'd call on Coralie this evening, on her way to work and she'd phone me about how she'd got on. She wanted me to tell Frankie that she hadn't been able to get anyone to do her duty so she'd have to give the party a miss.

'I don't know how long it'll take.' Mona said. 'But I'm sure to have news for you by about eight.'

Then could she phone me at Frankie's, I asked her, and she said yes, of course; it would probably be well before eight when there was news.

'And phone me anyway, whatever the result.' I said, a million doubts now raking me. Coralie might be out, although I knew this was unlikely. Far more likely that she wouldn't speak to Mona or slam the door in her face. Still, Mona was, in her own way, tougher than Coralie, and obviously, the way she'd sounded over the phone, shocked with anger that La Kane was bent on the destruction of someone like Oliver.

My imaginings were interrupted by Oliver. He looked grey and gaunt. The fact that he was functioning at all was really to his credit. 'Olwyn kept looking at me. I'm sure she suspects,' he groaned. 'She's not herself at all. You can't be married as long as we have without, well, a feeling that there's something wrong even though nothing's said. You don't think Coralie's been getting at Olwyn again, do you?' He was cracking his fingers with unnerving little reports.

To head him off surmises about Olwyn I told him of the plan with Mona. You never knew, it might work. Till we heard from Mona we'd both play dumb. But I had told Frankie, I said; I could never keep things from her.

'You warned her not to tell Olwyn?' he asked.

'Of course. All we can do now is try and contain ourselves till we hear from Mona.'

I must have looked pretty rough because several people expressed concern, especially Mr Latimer who was most solicitous. I could see he was nearly exploding with curiosity, especially as he told me that Doctor Stafford didn't seem himself either –he'd been quite snappy because one of the patients due for ECT couldn't have it because of eating breakfast. Usually Doctor Stafford would take something like that in his stride, Latimer said.

'But not today. Oh, no, he flew into a state and for the first time I thought him and me were going to have words. Is he in trouble, Doctor Delaney? There's a rumour going round that he and his wife are off to New Zealand?' Latimer was all concern.

Where had the New Zealand rumour started? I doubted whether it came from Mona; of course it was possible that Oliver had mentioned it himself. I told Latimer that too many good doctors were emigrating and it was probable that Doctor Stafford was considering it.

'Of course he's only a locum here,' I added.

Then I tried to change the subject by asking Latimer whether he had any work for me. But the ward was unusually quiet, half empty in fact and Doctor Stafford had attended to such problems as they had. It was the same on the other wards; Oliver was ahead of me mopping everything up although I would have welcomed something to do to take my mind off things, I was glad to have a clinic in the afternoon and I parried Morgan's anxious enquiries about whether I was feeling well.

'Sorry, but there's one patient who hasn't an appointment, Doctor,' Morgan said. 'A Barry Flount. He's terribly agitated and his wife is with him. She'd like to see you first.'

O.K., I said. I had nearly finished the clinic and though it was well after five o'clock I would make time for Barry. He was a hard driving company director who suffered from psychotic episodes, kept in control by long-acting injections of a psychotrophic drug which he had every two weeks. Unfortunately Barry reneged on these injections when business boomed or he had to travel to the EEC countries. And poor Mrs Flount was sick with worry today.

She was small and rather ugly but her very lovely greenish blue eyes had such dark circles under them that she looked like a bush baby. The weekend had been awful, she was afraid of her husband who had taken to fiddling with the gas fires and she thought he ought to come into hospital. I thought so, too, when he charged in. Normally amiable and gentle he was now suspiciously aggressive and so edgy that he kept jumping up and down and rambling on about pseudophilosophic matters, always a sign that he was ill. He was dirty and dishevelled looking with an unshaven face, and I knew he'd resent it when I told him that he needed to be in hospital.

'You've had a get-together with my wife, haven't you? Ganging up as usual.'

He jumped up and crashed his fists on the desk, so much was the force that the pile of patients' folders slid to the floor. Mrs Flount tried to get him to sit down again and he shouted, 'I know your little game. You want me put away again so you can be with your lover. Oh, yes, I'm on to you.'

He was roaring like a maddened animal and then he announced that he was going to drive to London as fast as he could. Mrs Flount turned ashen and I asked Barry please,

please to let his wife drive to him to the hospital. He turned at the door, face fixed and contorted and then he flung the keys at his wife. He came back to the table, his complexion now plum coloured, there were blobs of matter on the inside of his eyes and spittle trickled from his mouth. For a moment I thought he was going to strike me. He didn't, but his words rained on me like bullets from a well-aimed gun.

'Fucking woman. Sitting there telling everyone what to do. I bet you can't fucking manage your own life.'

Mrs Flount tried to say something, but I told her quickly to go after him, because he had rushed out, and that I was all right. But inside I felt a sort of sickness although I knew how mad Barry was, how unresponsible for what he said and did. His final screech of impotent rage underlined the fact that I seemed to have had more than my share of aggressive outbursts from patients. Coralie yesterday and Barry today. The sheer hatred of Barry's bellow of 'fucking woman' had the force of a blinding blow on the face.

I knew I'd better see to telling the hospital that he was on his way. Maybe Oliver was still around, although it was just after seven o'clock. I was put through to him in Gilbert Ward and he hardly let me finish about Barry Flount when he asked me whether I had heard from Mona. When I said no he sighed despairingly that it wouldn't work; Coralie had seemed utterly implacable. Maybe, but I'd bet that Mona was a match for her, I said.

I had forgotten my worry till now, especially with doing the clinic, but all my inner doubts were returning and I had to force myself into a cheerful manner. No news was good news. We hadn't heard that Mona had been unable to crack Coralie. Anyway, he was to let me know if Barry Flount failed to show up at the hospital and I'd see him at Frankie's. He said he'd come over as soon as he was finished in the hospital but could I give Olwyn a lift to Frankie's just in case? I said sure and wished I felt as jaunty as I sounded.

As I dressed to go to Frankie's I found myself tensed for

the phone. I was tired and jumpy and I kept dropping things and mislaying them. After I'd swept up a shattered scent bottle which had slipped from my clumsy fingers I went down for Olwyn.

'You do look nice,' I said.

And she did. She had washed her cloud of dark hair and used something, kohl probably, which accentuated her Modigliani-shaped eyes. Only someone of her fragile beauty could get away with the black shift dress she was wearing. She laughed and chattered all the way over, telling me how she was going to wear out all the few smart clothes she had because in a few months she wouldn't be able to. Poor Olwyn. Possibly we'd have done better to tell her, prevented her from mounting the big pink cloud she was obviously airborne on. We shouldn't have let her drift into a fantasy world which would have to be shattered when Mona drew a blank.

It was now five minutes past eight and I had heard nothing from Mona as I told Frankie when she seated Olwyn near Barney, who was playing Beethoven on the grand piano; Frankie had been pleased to hear about Olwyn's pregnancy but like me, after listening to my ploy with Mona, agreed that things were black and probably getting blacker.

'Poor little thing. The timing's so bloody wrong in life; she get's what she wants, what they both want, and at the same time there's the danger of her husband being disgraced. Anyway, you've done your best. We'll all just have to wait. It's only twenty past eight. Here . . .'

Frankie bent over the oven and brought out some small prawn vol au vents. She looked rather magnificent and had done her hair differently, it fell in a sort of cascade and her long silver earrings tinkled as she arranged the small eats on two plates.

'You take one . . .' She said, handing me a plate, 'and we'll both have an enormous drink.'

Barney had the same idea because when we came back to the sitting-room he was standing at the drinks table pouring himself a colossal whisky which Frankie tried to snatch from him. He made one of those deft avoidance movements he was so skilled at, and some of the drink splashed from the glass as he bellowed troumphantly that she could go to hell, she and all the other doctors he was drinking to forget about.

'You'll end up back in hospital.' Frankie shouted. It must have been the strain we were all feeling, her voice sounded carping and querulous. And Barney glowered at her; all the ingredients for battle were there. Wouldn't he play some more for us? I asked hastily. He used the piano so seldom, I went on and then seeking any way to divert him, I asked how it was that Beethoven composed so marvellously even though he'd been stone deaf?

'As if deafness precluded composing? Such rubbish.' Barney sniffed. But he went back to where Olwyn was waiting. She was all gentleness and composure tonight, probably a mixture of hormones and her own delight in her condition. Whatever it was she provided the ideal audience for Barney and, as I whispered to Frankie, we mustn't tell her about Oliver's troubles until we absolutely had to, and that would be soon enough, we decided looking at the clock which said twenty to nine. There was still hope, Frankie said. We had yet to hear that Mona hadn't been able to do anything. But she knew . . . and I knew . . . that Mona realised how worried we all were, so surely – if she had succeeded – she'd have given us news before this?

Though Frankie's voice was perky, her face was steeped in misery and we both sat in silence, unable to manufacture soothing clichés. So flattened was she that she couldn't even rise to the double bait of Barney remarking in a loud voice to Olwyn how strange it was that he couldn't hear a master like Beethoven, whilst Frankie's voice was stridently clear to him. Then he got up, looking defiantly at Frankie and poured himself another massive drink. In an effort to divert her, I told her how well Barney looked. So he did, he had all his old élan back but his neck was scraggy and the way his cheeks had fallen in made him look Punch-like in profile.

The clock hypnotised us. Olwyn was so entranced with Barney's sparkling interpretations on the piano that fortunately she didn't seem to notice how antisocial Frankie and I were. It was now after nine o'clock and no phone call, nothing at all from Mona.

When the door bell rang Frankie and I dashed out to the hall. For a wild moment I thought it was Mona. It was Oliver and he looked strained and sick. Barry Flount, he said was asleep. Usually Oliver wouldn't have left it at that about a patient. Not just a flat statement. He looked at us for news and I shook ny head. He shrugged hopelessly and we all three stared at each other. And there was the rest of the evening to be got through in some charade-like pretence that things weren't too bad. I didn't dare to think of having to break it to Olwyn, especially in her state of delight about being pregnant. Then the phone rang and I snatched it up. It was Mona.

'All is well. Coralie has withdrawn everything.' She sounded far away but I could just about hear what she said. 'Every call box was engaged,' she was saying. 'And when I got to the hospital a patient decided to have a cardiac arrest. Yes, she called me everything; I've learned a few variations on four letter words but the big thing is that she's beaten and withdrawing the allegations,' Mona said.

'You're a wonder and a marvel,' I said, overwhelmed. Oliver and Frankie were hugging each other and shouting that I was to thank Mona. 'Just a nasty thought,' I want on to Mona. 'Knowing the Kane psyche as I do, she might do a volte face. Change her mind in fact.'

'I thought of that, too,' Mona said and as usual I felt remiss in that I'd underestimated her again. 'I thought of that, so I got it in writing from Coralie. It took time, I've been ages I know, but I've got the retraction in writing. I'd better dash, somebody's drip has stuck.'

Frankie rushed off in quest of champagne and Oliver came to life. He stretched, sighed and visibly relaxed from his state of tension. He was sorry he had put me and everyone to such trouble and he wanted to thank me for my help. And to let me know that Olwyn and he were both of a mind to try New Zealand; but in the meantime he'd like to carry on working at Barrington.

'I suppose I'd better tell Olwyn,' he said.

I interposed quickly that that could wait. 'Don't tell her. Not tonight anyway. *She* has something to tell you,' I said.

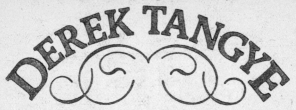

OFFICE LIFE

BY KEITH WATERHOUSE,
bestselling author of BILLY LIAR

OFFICE BUREAUCRACY LAID BARE!

From the ranks of the nation's clerks, Clement Gryce has surfaced from redundancy to join the working force at British Albion. The Stationery Supplies department on the seventh floor is Gryce's new billet and his colleagues – particularly the lovely Miss Divorce – seem just the ticket. Duties are light, not to say minimal.

Even so, there's something strange about British Albion. What does the company actually do? Why don't the telephones ever ring? Why does Lucas of Personnel make mysterious enquiries about Gryce's political beliefs? And why are two entire floors devoted to issuing luncheon vouchers for the staff canteen? The suspense is too much for Gryce, he decides the matter needs investigation and sets forth on a voyage of discovery all his own . . .

Anyone who has ever worked in the world of 'top-copy-and-two-carbons' will recognize the lunacies of office bureaucracy laid bare in this brilliantly savage lampoon.

And don't miss Keith Waterhouse's hilarious novel
JUBB
also available in Sphere Books

GENERAL FICTION   0 7221 0522 3   £1.25